The 9 Principles for a Lean and Defined Body

By Philip J. Hoffman M.S., MBA
Body Transformation Coach
Fit-Lifestyle Model
Author

Contents

Part Two

Appendices

Preface

My name is Philip Hoffman, founder of *HoffmanFit Lean Body System*.

Obesity isn't a small problem our nation faces today; it's an epidemic. The hundreds of diet and fitness programs that flood the market with fad bestselling books, late-night infomercials, and "magic pills" are only making the problem worse. So why is it that millions of Americans aren't able to maintain a healthy body weight?

First, because the challenge of losing body fat—especially belly fat around the waistline—is an issue of practicing consistent, long-term healthy eating habits that are sustainable for the rest of your life.

Second, because most people have no idea which type of workouts are actually the most effective for losing body fat.

The HoffmanFit Lean Body System is a no-nonsense muscle-building and fat-loss system. My system is sustainable and meant to be practiced as a lifestyle rather than a short term solution. Because of the sustainability, you don't have to think about how to manage your weight ever again. This results-driven system incorporates nine critical principles:

1) Follow a simplified and sustainable system
2) Train with weights to build muscle
3) Learn proper exercise form and technique
4) Train at a high-intensity level to stimulate muscle growth
5) Forget everything you've learned about health & fitness
6) Nutritional habits contribute 80% to your results
7) Processed foods are like addictive drugs
8) There is no magic pill—only correct information on which to act
9) Organize your environment to maintain order in your life

These principles were developed from my personal experience as a competitive bodybuilder and fitness model, 10+ years of academic studies in the biological and nutritional sciences, and, more importantly, feedback from hundreds of clients with whom I've spent thousands of hours consulting with on muscle-building and fat-burning strategies.

Applying each principle in this book is crucial to your success. They aren't rules of a "quick fix" program; they're proven principles that, when applied, will increase the quality of your overall health and body shape more than anything else you could do.

Here's a fact: six-pack abs and flat stomachs aren't achieved without high levels of fitness and low levels of body fat—which is why very few people ever achieve them. The problem is, most people are working out using incorrect strategies that don't produce expected results. *The HoffmanFit Lean Body System* changes all of this; this will be specifically demonstrated in my newest book, *HD Six-Pack Abs, The Art & Science to a Flat and Defined Set of Abs*, which will release in 2015.

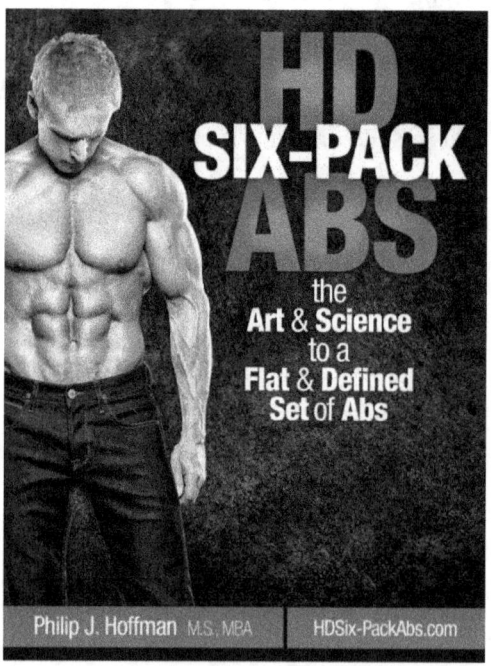

Your health is, by far, the most important part and greatest asset of your life. It's important that whomever you trust with it is not only educated in the biological sciences, but can also provide you with safe, effective methods that have your best interests at heart. Why trust me? I've devoted my life to the study and practice of health, exercise, and nutrition—particularly focusing on the development of muscle and the regulation of body fat and metabolism. At 50+ years old, I'm in the best shape of my life and have significantly slowed the biological aging process down to that of someone two decades younger.

As you read this book, allow me to be your personal coach—the person who helps monitor the validity, quality, and effectiveness of the messages being thrown at you from the health and fitness industry. As an authority on fitness and nutrition, I stay constantly up to date with the latest peer-reviewed research in the industry (rather than "garbage science," which is what I call the nonobjective research that supplement companies conduct for their own benefit).

The *HoffmanFit Lean Body System* encompasses everything I've learned and experienced in the realm of personal health and fitness. It was created with a sense of artistry and experience—not just a mass of scientific knowledge—to make it the most powerful, results-driven program in the industry.

Are you ready to be in the best shape and health of your life?

Let's get started.

Principle 1:
Create a Simplified and Sustainable System and Follow It

Develop a scientifically sound, effective, and sustainable plan of action that includes exercise and healthy eating.

MAKE A PLAN

No goal can be achieved without a plan to back it up. Whether you want to be the next top surgeon, athlete, or business professional, you must implement a strategic system that guides you to each goal you set. The same idea must be applied to your health and fitness goals.

Take the time to develop, write down, and then practice a health and fitness plan that fits your lifestyle, and is something you can stick to for the long haul.

Tracking the small activities—whether it's the food you're eating or the exercises you're completing each day—is critical in reaching your bigger goal. You don't need to rely on someone else to keep you accountable; you need to keep *yourself* accountable. Practice it, live by it, and make it habitual. I've posted sample food tracking and exercise tracking sheets here on my website to help you get your start.

Tracking progress: It's what winners do.

HAVE REALISTIC EXPECTATIONS

One of the easiest ways to fail is by creating an unrealistic daily routine that won't fit your lifestyle. If you know you won't wake up at 5:30 in the morning to work out, don't plan on it in your routine.

Another easy way to fail is by harboring false expectations about how you can transform your body in a quick and easy manner. The amount of information that's fed to us through health and fitness TV shows, "blockbuster" diet books, and late-breaking "scientific" reports is enough to make anyone's head spin. Not sure what you can believe?

You're not alone. Maybe at one point you felt so bombarded and confused by conflicts in information that you quit before you even began—or maybe you lost twenty pounds on Weight Watchers only to eventually gain it back and try again on the South Beach Diet.

You may have heard of an individual who lost 30 pounds in 30 days on an all-fish-and-green-tea diet. Listen up: those diets aren't realistic, and they aren't going to do anything but harm your metabolism and overall health. I don't make any false promises to you about instant results with the *HoffmanFit Lean Body System.* Your return on this investment into your body will pay off at the right time in the right way.

You won't fit into your pair of skinny jeans next week.

JUDGE THE MERITS OF A PROGRAM

Never buy a new car without reading the reports on it, never open an email that says you just won a free Caribbean Cruise in the subject line, and never start a new fitness and nutrition program without analyzing it for its merits and long-term sustainability. If it's a "lose 10 pounds in two weeks" program you're interested in, don't bother. Those who do want a program like that will not do well with *HoffmanFit.* What happens when those two weeks are over? You're much better off avoiding the short-term fixes entirely when your chances of long-term failure are so high. Don't allow yourself to be lured in to the "fix-it" diets that will actually set you further back in your goals in the long run. There's no such thing as a free lunch—you must pay your dues to get something that's worth anything.

> Each time you begin a restrictive eating program to rapidly lose weight, your metabolism is further damaged. Your body actually becomes *more* efficient at storing fat. Isn't that the complete opposite of your goal?

As you determine the merits of any fitness program, here are the criteria that must be met:

1) The program should be based on scientifically sound, unbiased information
2) The program should include both exercise *and* a nutritional component
3) The exercises should consist mostly of full-body strength and conditioning training that incorporates the use of free weights
4) The intensity of the training must be high enough to stimulate muscular growth and development with sufficient weight to cause micro-tears to the muscle fibers.
5) The nutritional component should consider a macronutrient (proteins, carbs, fats) ratio and calorie reduction to cause fat loss while sparing lean muscle tissue.
6) The program should not consider the use of *any* supplement as a means of contributing to results.
7) The program should emphasize consistency and repetition of its fundamental principles to produce maximum results.
8) The program should avoid the useless, confusing diet-related details and minutiae commonly published by the media
9) The program can be easily implemented and followed by anyone

If you follow *HoffmanFit*, no damage to your metabolism can occur. I've created a lifestyle program, *not* a "fix-it" diet, that takes all of the important components of your health into consideration. I told you that I wouldn't make you any false promises, and I won't. Here's what I can guarantee about my program:

1) You *will* get strong, lean, and fit to achieve your best body possible
2) You *will* be following a program that meets all the criteria listed above
3) You *will* be following a program that can be practiced for the rest of your life

DON'T RELY ON ANYONE BUT YOURSELF

Workout buddies or accountability partners can be a valuable asset to have—but they can just as easily be a hindrance to your progress.

Buddying up with someone reduces your need to take total responsibility for reaching your goals.

"Susie can't run today? I'll just stay home, then. We'll go tomorrow."

"Bob can't make our weekly racquetball game? I could stay late at the office tonight."

"Liz called in a cheat day to enjoy some chocolate cake and take a break from working out? I might as well join her; we'll work it off tomorrow."

See what happens?

Over the years I've learned to keep control of the outcome of my own personal plan by solely assuming the responsibility of my actions. If the other person encounters a personal problem and can't continue the same activities with you, how will you respond to the change? Only depend on *yourself* in these situations where your best interests are at stake.

Develop the mindset that **you and only you** are responsible for the outcome of your decisions, behavior and habits. Don't allow room for any excuses.

If you can find someone who is truly as committed as you, and you're someone that becomes more motivated by working with a partner, then absolutely partner up. But be aware—there's nothing more disappointing than hearing someone make excuses for why they could not accomplish a goal due to another person's actions.

Make it clear to each other that excuses are not acceptable.

PERSONALIZE YOUR WORKOUT SCHEDULE

In order to maximize your workout experience, my recommendation is to follow a schedule that allows you to work out as many days per week as possible. Ultimately, that means six days per week; minimally, four days per week. Don't be concerned about overtraining because my programs provide proper recovery between muscle groups. I'm a proponent of working out every day because it helps to form good fitness habits. The more a behavior becomes a habit, the harder it is to break that habit and the easier it becomes to perform that activity.

I see so many people at the gym aimlessly walking around without a systematic workout program that will produce results. This is a huge cause of failure, and why so many people become frustrated because they don't experience results from their efforts.

You must have a system and schedule to follow that includes:

- which days and what hour you'll work out
- which muscle groups you'll train each workout
- which exercises you'll perform for each workout

For now, it's important to understand that it's crucial to have a program that leads to the achievement of your goals.

Action Steps Principle 1

Goal: Practice regular fitness and nutrition habits by incorporating the* HoffmanFit *principles.

- Buy a journal and analyze your schedule. Can you remove one current activity and replace it with another? I don't recommend sudden, drastic changes for everyone. After you finish reading this book, choose the principles you want to start with first and then add more as you become more comfortable. If you're an all-or-nothing kind of person like me, then do it.
- Determine where in your schedule you can free-up about four to six, 30- to 45-minute sessions per week for the exercise portion of my system. Allow time to travel to the gym as well.
- Find time for two supermarket shopping and prepping sessions during the week for purchasing, cleaning, preparing, cooking and storing food items for all of your meals. Instead of cooking one meal at a time for you and your family, you'll be preparing food

for several meals. This alone will save you hours of time if you're currently cooking and cleaning for a family on a daily basis. You will need approximately two hours per session for a total of four hours per week to prepare your meals in advance. (I will discuss this more in the Nutrition chapter of Part Two in this book).

You might be thinking this seems like a lot of time. If so, then consider the time it takes to prepare one meal at a time—as well as the cleaning involved after each meal—versus implementing my food prep system. Or, try adding up the time it takes to go to a restaurant, wait for your food, and drive home each time you dine out. Still think it's too much time?

These practices create a sensible, sustainable lifestyle that meets all the Principle 1 criteria.

> We make bad decisions when we're stressed and rushed. Ideally, the total time needed to implement the full course of action (the workouts, shopping, food prep, and clean up) is approximately **eight hours per week.**

Think about it this way: if we break down the eight hours per week that you invest in your health and look at this on a daily basis, it comes down to 75 minutes. That's slightly more than an hour a day. Not bad when you consider this includes both the exercise *and* the nutrition components of my system.

Now you need to ask yourself, are there 75 minutes throughout the day where I could replace an activity that contributes nothing significant to my life (such as watching TV or surfing the internet) with an activity that will be enhance my quality of life like being fit and looking and feeling great?

I believe you can find the time if it's important enough.

Principle 2:
Build Muscle with Weight Training

---

*Train with weights to increase lean muscle, burn fat, shape
the body, and increase your metabolism 24/7.*

BUILD MUSCLE, INCREASE YOUR METABOLISM

Weight training—specifically with free weights, not exercise machines—will help you build lean muscle more than any other training method available. In order to build muscle, there must be enough of a stimulus on each muscle fiber to result in break-down or tearing of the fibers, followed by a subsequent rest or growth period.

This phenomenon occurs to a greater extent with weight training than with any other training method. This doesn't mean other training methods aren't beneficial, but it's a fact that lean muscle tissue is developed to a much greater degree through resistance training with weights.

One of the important goals in combating the aging process is to preserve muscle tissue and prevent **muscle atrophy**, or the wasting of tissue. **Sarcopenia** is the loss of skeletal muscle tissue due to the aging process, during which muscle tissue is replaced by fat—whereby the metabolic rate severely declines. Since the aging process brings loss of muscle mass and a subsequent slowing of the metabolism, it makes sense to engage in the type of training that preserves the greatest amount of muscle mass.

Lean muscle tissue is metabolically active tissue because it possesses the sub-cellular organelle called the **mitochondria**. These structures are where cell respiration occurs; therefore, more lean muscle tissue = increased number of mitochondria = increased resting metabolic rate. That means your body burns more calories even while you're not performing physical activity.

Benefits of Weight Training

If you want a strong, shapely, and healthy body, consistent weight training is a must. In addition to preventing sarcopenia, weight training provides countless other benefits. Here are just a few of them:

1) *Women* – Females can benefit even more from weight training than males. Since the female endocrine system has endowed women with a different set of hormones, the struggle to keep body fat levels in check is significantly more difficult. Lifting weights to increase lean muscle, in my opinion, is the most important activity a female can do. By developing a higher percentage of muscle earlier in life, the inevitable loss of muscle tissue due to aging can be slowed. Weight training can also thwart osteoporosis, which many females encounter after menopause.

2) *Sculpting* – We are our body's own sculptor. Weight training is the ultimate tool for creating shape, developing curves, and chiseling your body. Plastic surgery can't hold a candle to the results you can get from weight training.

3) *Motivation* – Nothing is more motivating than transforming your body with weights and proper eating habits. The appearance of a muscular physique exudes confidence and self-control—not to mention the admiration it garners from others.

FORGET LONG CARDIO SESSIONS: THE AEROBIC HOAX

How often have you been told to "perform 30- to 60-minute sessions of steady cardio three to five times per week," and to "stay in your fat-burning zone?" For the past couple of decades we've been told that aerobic exercise is the best way to burn calories and fat. You may be surprised to learn how little those cardio sessions actually benefit you.

The most recent research shows that short bursts of high-intensity drills are much more effective for developing a lean, muscular body versus low-intensity, steady movements. The best example of this can be seen with sprinters and marathon runners. Sprinters have very lean and muscular physiques, while marathon runners often have an emaciated, weak appearance.

The whole idea of maintaining a lean body is to keep as much muscle tissue as possible. Long cardio sessions burn calories only during the exercise session while short, high-intensity training helps develop lean muscle tissue long after the exercise session has ended.

Since muscle tissue is the metabolically active tissue in the body, the real benefit—in terms of burning calories—comes from the extra calories burned throughout the day. This phenomenon of calories burned hours after completing the exercise session is called **the "after-burn effect."** Nobody knows the exact number of additional calories burned, but estimates are about 15% more than by not weight training.

There is even strong evidence suggesting that long cardio sessions can actually be unhealthy. Not only can that type of training cause excessive damage to the tendons, ligaments, and joints of the body, but it also can result in cellular damage through the production of free radicals. Note: I'm strictly referring to individuals that run many miles per week and compete in long-distance running—not the occasional runner logging a couple miles each day.

Another commonly debated argument is that of conditioning the heart and lungs to reduce the resting heart rate. There is no evidence or rule proving long cardio sessions are the only means of reducing resting heart rates. In fact, high-intensity resistance training results in conditioning of the heart and lungs because it includes training with short rest periods to keep the heart rate elevated. I personally have a low resting heart rate in the range of 58 beats per minute (bpm), yet have rarely done any cardio training in over 25 years.

Action Steps: Principle 2

Goal: Find a good gym or invest in free weights for your home.
16

During Principle 1 action steps, we discussed scheduling four to six time periods of 30-45 minutes each week to start training. Now that you know the truth about long, slow cardio sessions, I recommend filling those 30-45 minute sessions with exercises that incorporate free weights—specifically with dumbbells—and high-intensity resistance training, whether your workout takes place at the gym or at home.

For extensive information on whether a fitness club or home gym is the right environment for you, refer to the Workout Chapter in Part Two of this book.

Principle 3:
Learn Proper Exercise Form and Technique

Perform exercise movements correctly through a full range of motion with appropriate size weights to fully develop and properly shape your muscles.

DON'T OVERDO IT

After 30+ years of training in countless gyms and health clubs all over the world, I've had the chance to observe the workout habits of thousands of workout enthusiasts... and yet I don't believe that many of them have made significant muscular improvements.

We can reasonably assume gym goers want to progress, whether by building muscle, losing body fat, or getting stronger—likely a combination of the three. We can also reasonably assume these individuals desire to make the most of their efforts by executing proper exercise form and technique.

But that's not what I've been observing over time.

Many workout enthusiasts—particularly males—fail to make significant progress because they perform the exercise movement incorrectly; they often try to lift weights that are too heavy, and their desire to impress those around them gets in the way of practicing proper form. The full range of motion is significantly reduced, so the muscle is cheated of complete stimulation of its fibers. This, in turn, decreases the tearing down of the microfibers within the muscle in order for the re-building phase to take place during the healing process. As a consequence, muscle hypertrophy doesn't occur nearly to the extent that it would if proper exercise form were executed.

In this sense, progress is less than optimal due to one's ego. By being more concerned with the appearance of looking strong, many people sabotage and delay their muscular gains rather than reaping the rewards by using a lighter, more controllable weight.

Your muscles don't know what size weights you are using.

What they *do* respond to is the resistance or force generated against the muscle. One might argue that the heavier the weight, the higher the number of muscle fibers being stimulated—resulting in the greatest muscle development. Theoretically, this can be true as long as the exercise is being executed along a full range of motion—in perfect form.

However, the problem lies within the execution of the exercise.

Rarely do individuals pay enough attention to the form of their exercise movements. As I said earlier, the heavier the weights used, the more your exercise form is compromised; thus, your muscles are cheated of their full potential.

Muscles are blind to the number appearing on the side of the dumbbell or barbell; instead, muscle responds to the principle of **time under tension (TUT).** For example, I can perform an exercise set with a heavier than normal weight and pump out 10 repetitions while ignoring my form. But if I perform another set with a lighter weight and execute perfect form through a full range of motion, I will stimulate a much higher number of fibers, leading to much greater muscular development.

LIST OF PRIMARY EXERCISES

Below, I've listed a variety of 15 effective exercises which work the entire body. These exercises were selected specifically because they shape and define every muscle group and help stimulate the release of your fat-burning hormones to the highest degree.

The exercises may seem overwhelming in the beginning, but they will feel easier as you become familiar with the movements. I recommend you go to the link on my website provided below and view each exercise along with its respective description to become more familiar.

Legs	Dumbbell (DB) or Goblet squats	Romanian dead-lifts	DB lunges
Back	Wide-grip pull downs	Bent-over DB rows	Pull-ups (assisted)
Chest	Flat bench DB press	Incline DB press	
Shoulders	DB shoulder press	DB side raises	Upright Rows
Triceps	Skull crushers	Cable pressdowns	
Biceps	Standing barbell curls		
Abdominals	Bicycle crossovers	Swiss ball crunches	

Action Steps: Principle 3

Goal: Perform each repetition with a complete range of motion and perfect technique.

Even after all my years of experience, I still find myself needing reminders from time to time that this is a lifestyle, not a temporary fitness program. We'll get to the details in later chapters, but for now, let's focus on the principle concepts.

In addition to the link to my tutorial page on my website, I've provided illustrations of each of the 19 exercises included in the table above along with a full description on how to properly perform the movement. You can find the exercises in Appendix C.

http://www.hoffmanfit.com/hoffman/tutorials/#E47

Here are some tips:

1) *Don't* get sloppy. Choose a dumbbell that allows you to perform each exercise movement with perfect execution.

2) *Don't* perform partial movements. Make sure that each repetition you perform is completed through a full range of motion.

3) *Do* feel slightly fatigued. What is the best size dumbbell for you? The one that allows you to fully complete 8-10 repetitions. If you're struggling, decrease the weight. If you're performing 8-10 repetitions without feeling fatigued, increase the weight a bit. To figure out what poundages you should start with, see the chart I've created in the "Workouts" section of Part Two of this book.

Principle 4:
Stimulate Muscle Growth with High-Intensity Training

Reduce gym time by training at high-intensity levels to maximize muscle growth and increase fat-burning hormones as well as your basal metabolic rate (BMR). Short rest periods between sets are key for muscle growth.

GYM TIME: QUALITY OVER QUANTITY

The *volume of work* completed during a workout session is where your focus should be—don't get hung up on how much time your workout takes to complete.

$$W = F \: x \: D$$

Work = Force x Distance

What does this equation mean? F (force) is the amount of weight moved with any exercise. This is multiplied by D (distance), meaning that the amount of work increases as either the force increases or the distance of the weight increases.

Simply put, the intensity of the workout increases as the amount of work increases in a given period of time. Make sense?

The flip side of this equation is even more important to be aware of:

> Taking long rests between exercises while using incorrect exercise form will completely derail your efforts for developing muscle.

The bottom line is: the amount of time you spend in the gym is irrelevant.

The amount of work completed during the exercise session is what matters. In order to effectively develop shapely muscles and increase your resting metabolic rate, it's important to complete the greatest amount of work in the shortest period of time. This is referred to as **high-intensity resistance training** (HIRT).

HIRT is absolutely crucial in developing muscle and creating a lean body. HIRT is well known for increasing muscle tissue, but not as much with fat-burning—until recently. HIRT is the most effective way to increase the amount of energy you burn at rest, referred to as your **basal metabolic rate** (BMR) and your **exercise post-oxygen consumption** (EPOC), or the after-burn effect.

Let's put this in English.

BMR is important because it tells us how many calories our body burns while at rest. Burning more calories at rest means you're burning fat at a faster rate. The more muscle tissue, the higher the BMR.

EPOC is the increased rate of oxygen intake following strenuous exercise. So if you walk up a flight of stairs, your oxygen rate automatically increases in response to strenuous movement. You don't tell your body what to do…it just knows.

Now imagine you are working out strenuously at the gym. Your body automatically responds to the need for more oxygen. This means that working out using HIRT principles can increase overall metabolism by about 15%. Since EPOC occurs 24/7 without you having to do anything extra to "kick it into gear," incorporating HIRT into your workout routine is wise.

Your EPOC factor—how quickly your metabolism returns to your BMR after exercise—is also important. Working out at a high-intensity level means your metabolism remains elevated for an extended period of time after you've completed your workout. This means you'll burn fat faster—hence, more fat loss!

HIRT FAVORABLY ALTERS YOUR HORMONE PROFILE

HIRT not only increases your BMR and EPOC, but also alters specific metabolic hormones in a favorable way.

Testosterone

Testosterone is the prominent hormone of muscular development. The release of testosterone occurs when muscle tissue is stimulated via weight training; that, in turn, causes structural changes within muscle—resulting in growth. In addition to its effects on protein synthesis, testosterone may also indirectly stimulate the release of **growth hormone** (GH).

Growth Hormone

GH is another powerful hormone that causes muscle tissue growth, or **anabolism**. Not only does GH promote muscular growth, but it's also involved in increasing **lipolysis**—the breaking down of fat. Though not fully understood, GH is also known to stimulate the release of insulin-like growth factors (IGFs) that increase the availability of **amino acids**—the building blocks of proteins for protein synthesis which results in greater tissue repair and growth.

Epinephrine/Norepinephrine

Another group of metabolic hormones released during intense weight training are the catecholamines **epinephrine and norepinephrine**—more commonly known as **adrenaline and noradrenaline**, respectively. These hormones are thought to inhibit the release of insulin, therefore preventing fat storage and having potentially extraordinary effects on fat loss. They are also very responsive to high-intensity training with very short rest periods between sets. Research has indicated these hormones can increase to more than 20 times that of resting levels. The body becomes more efficient at burning fat by learning how to manipulate these fat-burning hormones. Individuals can experience a 50-80% increase in the amount of fat that's mobilized from fat stores by working out at high-intensity levels.

Since muscle development and fat burning are the primary objectives, understanding how to control testosterone and GH is crucial to getting lean. To stimulate these hormones, large muscle group exercises must be performed using heavy enough weights and at a high enough intensity level to stimulate the breakdown of the maximum amount of muscle tissue.

If you are a beginner striving to gain lean muscle, these are the exercises you should be focusing on:

- Bench press
- Squats (DBs in hand)
- Romanian dead lifts
- Lunges
- Bent-over DB rows
- Shoulder press
- Pull-ups (assisted)
- Cable pressdowns or dips
- Standing barbell curls

In order to stimulate the release of the greatest amount of your body's natural anabolic hormones, my recommendation is to perform sets in the range of 8-10 repetitions. This is the range in which the vast majority of athletes train for muscular gains.

The bottom line is: in order to receive the full benefit of altering your hormone profile and increase your BMR, it is crucial to apply the principle of HIRT in all your workouts.

Action Step: Principle 4

Goal: Work out with a high level of intensity and minimal rest periods

Make sure to perform exercises at a high level of intensity during every workout. That means having rest periods of less than one minute between each set of exercises. For certain body parts such as arms, chest, and shoulders, rest periods will be even shorter than other muscle groups like legs. Leg exercises such as squats can require longer rest than upper body movements because they strongly stimulate the cardiovascular system and elevate your heart rate.

Principle 5:
Forget Everything You Know about Health & Fitness

Clear your mind of pre-conceived notions about building muscle, losing fat, and eating healthy. Learn the correct scientific principles that govern human physiology, and stop being deceived by the misleading information and scams so prevalent in the fitness and weight loss industry.

AVOID BEING DUPED

You've heard countless amounts of information on how to lose body fat, why you should take nutritional supplements, how you can develop muscle and build a six-pack, and the "truth" about all sorts of nutrition.

Forget it all.

Let's start this chapter with a clean slate and wipe our preconceived notions about what it takes to develop a lean, muscular body. I can tell you from experience that the most challenging part of my job is spending time and energy dispelling false and harmful information. In fact, I could go as far as to say that I've been unable to help a significant number of clients because their mind isn't capable of letting go of false beliefs such as "spot-reducing" for fat loss.

No industry causes more confusion than the health and fitness industry. Deception and downright lying is the norm for much of the weight loss and nutritional supplement markets. What *is* important is having a basic knowledge of human physiology, anatomy, and biochemistry in order to understand how the human body functions.

The nutritional supplement industry is, essentially, an unregulated industry that is to blame for much of the false advertising in the market. Manufacturers' claims about product results are misleading because no supporting objective scientific studies are required. In many instances, customer testimonies are the only elements of proof needed for supplement manufacturers to make the claims they do for product labels.

The real damage? Most people fail to make progress. Believing results can be achieved with a certain supplement, a trendy diet program, or a special piece of equipment deceives people into buying products that provide no value to the consumer. Even worse, an *enormous* amount of valuable time is wasted in an effort to get fit, lose weight, and become healthy.

How many times have you heard people talk about the numerous programs they've tried in hopes of getting fit and losing weight? The rollercoaster ride never ends! They're successful for a few months, only to gain back more weight than they started with after the ride is finished.

Remember this statistic:

95% of people that engage in a weight loss program don't keep the weight off longer than 12 months. Be part of the 5% *who do*.

ANYONE CAN PROVIDE MISINFORMATION—EVEN YOUR DOCTOR

It's very difficult to find valuable, quality information. If you're not armed with a good scam detector, it's almost impossible to distinguish the truth from the lies. You've been a victim of the industry and their biased opinions because they're selling a product that promises to change your body.

Don't be a victim any longer.

Be careful—even your medical doctor is not exempt from providing false information. Be cautious in seeking advice from your doctor on the subject of fitness and nutrition because he or she is probably not educated or informed on the subject unless they've taken a special interest in doing so. Most physicians receive only a few hours of nutritional education. There's even a good chance that your doctor still advises patients according to one of the biggest research blunders ever pulled on society called the **Lipid Hypothesis**.

The Lipid Hypothesis states that high blood cholesterol increases the risk of heart disease, and that reducing cholesterol reduces this risk. This hypothesis—now debunked—has led millions of people to avoid saturated fats from certain foods such as animal products. This 35-year-old myth has perpetuated a misunderstanding of the relationship between lipids, fats, and cholesterol to heart disease—yet many physicians haven't changed the way they treat patients despite the revelation of this blunder.

The popular thinking is that reducing the level of plasma cholesterol will reduce one's risk of suffering a new coronary heart disease event. The fact that people with higher plasma cholesterol levels suffer coronary heart disease at younger ages is undisputed. However, this premise has not yet been proved true to the satisfaction of research scientists, or of the medical community at large. The Lipid Hypothesis, then, is simply an inference derived from accepted facts.

Unfortunately, mainstream medicine is greatly influenced by the pharmaceutical industry, which makes a huge amount of money on cholesterol-lowering drugs called statins. It's therefore in the industry's financial interest to perpetuate these myths and continue exerting their enormous influence on doctors.

By rethinking all the myths you've been taught, you'll be less likely to fall victim to the unscrupulous marketers of products and services for the fitness and weight loss industry in the future. You'll also start to learn valuable information that will help you achieve your goals.

More importantly, you'll start to take *personal responsibility* for your health.

DON'T FUSS OVER SMALL THINGS

Many individuals in the fitness and weight loss industry constantly focus on small and trivial details—minutiae—that ultimately don't matter in achieving your fitness goals.

"Is it better to work out in the morning or evening?"

"Should I eat organic lettuce? I heard pesticides can make you fat."

"Should I avoid all carbs to lose more fat?"

"Should I lift light weights and do extra reps to prevent getting bulky?"

"Should I eat six meals a day to keep my metabolism higher?"

These aren't the important questions. So why do we ask them? It's because we are overwhelmed with confusing and contradictory information. When we are confused, we procrastinate. Often, focusing on the minutiae is used as a mental tactic to stall time before being forced to take action. People who worry about the little things are generally not the people who are working out, eating healthy, and achieving great results.

Worrying about trivial details is a waste of time. Put an end to it!

ACT ONLY ON PROVEN INFORMATION

I don't teach principles that I don't personally practice every day. Why would you believe in someone's program if the person preaching the program can't achieve the success he or she is claiming it can achieve? I'm a huge believer of this.

See the chapter in the second half of this book titled "Workouts & Training for the 40+ population: Boomer-itis" for recent photos of me and updates on my health status at 50+ years old. Since I'm often asked about using performance enhancing drugs, I've put this issue to rest by subjecting myself to an Anabolic Steroid test at the same time this photo was taken to prove a point. If interested, you can review the results on my website:

http://www.hoffmanfit.com/TestresultsHoffmanP.pdf

Action Step: Principle 5

Goal: Take time to educate yourself. Learn the real facts about fitness and nutrition.

Don't believe in something solely because the 3 a.m. infomercial you watched says it works and offers a money-back guarantee. This is what's referred to as **anecdotal evidence**. Unfortunately, anecdotal evidence is often accepted in lieu of solid scientific evidence. Whenever possible, seek peer-reviewed scientific evidence when looking at anything supplement-related. Working with legitimate, science-supported information is one of the most important keys to achieving your goals.

Principle 6:
Nutritional Habits Contribute Nearly 80% to Results

Focus primarily on nutritional habits for fat loss. Then learn how to implement a system of purchasing, preparing, cooking, and storing a core list of healthy foods in advance for quick and tasty meals.

GET YOUR FACTS STRAIGHT ON NUTRITION

"I have to get back to the gym to start losing weight!"

How many times have you heard this—from a friend's mouth or your own? I've heard it hundreds of times from clients who believe a personal trainer can solve their weight issues. Unfortunately, simply joining a gym or working with a trainer rarely has much of an effect on fat loss.

Here's why this is true: working out and maintaining proper nutritional habits contribute differently to the overall goal of developing a lean and muscular body. You can't achieve leanness without good nutritional habits, and you can't gain muscle without working out.

Before you even begin a nutritional program, you *must* understand nutrition and food choice basics. Ultimately, it's the total calories consumed daily that determine your weight and body fat levels. Sounds like I'm stating the obvious, right? You'd be surprised how many people have been misled into thinking that calories don't matter. They've been taught that if you don't consume carbohydrates, for example, then total calories don't matter. Nothing could be further from the truth.

"Is a calorie a calorie?" That's the million dollar question in nutrition and weight loss. In other words, does it matter the source of the calorie, or are all calories the same? Is 100 calories of chocolate cake the same as 100 calories of broccoli? The truth is that *both* total calories and the source of those calories matter when trying to reduce body fat.

All foods contain calories, and all calories consist of the macronutrients: **proteins, carbohydrates, and fats**. Some foods provide calories from protein, like eggs and chicken breast, while other foods contribute more calories from fats, like avocados or peanut butter.

Simplified Diagram Of Breakdown Of Calories

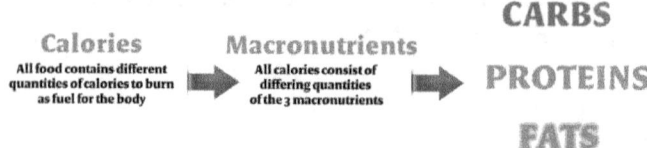

Calories
All food contains different quantities of calories to burn as fuel for the body

Macronutrients
All calories consist of differing quantities of the 3 macronutrients

CARBS

PROTEINS

FATS

All foods consist of differing quantities of carbohydrates, protein and fats

You need all three macronutrients for a healthy, functioning body. Understanding calories and carbohydrates is where most people become confused.

Many people are misled to believe that by not consuming carbohydrates, they will automatically lose weight. Although the American diet consists of disproportionate percentages of processed or refined carbohydrates from fast foods, sugar, flour, white rice, cereals, wheat products, crackers, salad dressings, chips, and pasta, avoiding these sources of food will *not* guarantee weight loss.

The reason why carbs are vilified and targeted as responsible for the obesity epidemic is because most of the carbs consumed and discussed in the media are **processed or refined carbs** (what we don't want), rather than **complex carbs** (what we *do* want). This misunderstanding has resulted in a great disservice to public health since all types of carbs are often grouped together and therefore totally avoided in the diets of many individuals.

Rather than eliminate one of the three macronutrients—carbs, in this case—it makes more sense to consider the total calories consumed from all three of the macronutrients. The total number of calories you consume on a daily basis is the most important factor in determining loss of body fat and getting lean. It's the first factor I consider when reviewing a client's nutritional profile before looking at anything else.

If you consume an extra 1200 calories a day, even if you've cut most carbs out of your diet, you'll *still* gain weight. Carbohydrates alone don't make you fat; generally speaking, too many calories are what make you fat—regardless of the source.

> Eating excess healthy food still results in consuming a surplus of calories which violates the calorie deficit rule for fat loss.

Once you have a correct understanding of the three macronutrients that make up a calorie, other topics in nutrition become easier to understand. I explain this in more detail in Part Two of this book. This is especially helpful when you make food choices at the supermarket, and when you start to estimate your total daily caloric intake and breakdown of your macronutrient ratio.

PREPARE FOOD IN ADVANCE FOR QUICK MEALS

Time is our most precious commodity. Adding regular exercise, grocery shopping, and food preparation for a family can be time-consuming to schedules already tight with activity. But something has to give in order to solve the shortage of time, right?

My focus in developing my *HoffmanFit Lean Body System* was and always will be on saving valuable time for my clients. I developed a system that decreases the time involved with shopping, preparing, storing, and cooking healthy meals. I don't like wasting time, so I've created an efficient system for preparing healthy food by carefully timing all the events involved with the process. Of course, as life changes I am constantly searching for new ways of improving it.

Leaving things "up in the air" isn't a good practice for being successful at anything. Every day, when I go to the gym, I've already decided which muscle group I'm training and which exercises I'll be performing. This same idea applies to meal planning. The evening before, I remove certain food items from the freezer and make sure I'm not missing an item from the supermarket for the next day's meals.

The best time-saving strategy is to prepare food in advance so that healthy meals can be prepared and ready to eat in 10 minutes or less. This solves two important issues: having more time and eating healthy.

I don't leave *anything* to chance. My program saves hours of time and hundreds of dollars each month; it's very healthy, and I honestly enjoy every part of the process. If you make advanced meal preparation a habit, I guarantee you'll enjoy having a sustainably healthy and energy-boosting lifestyle.

SHOP FROM A CORE LIST OF FOODS

You don't need to attend culinary school to learn how to prepare meals.

In fact, chef-created meals are often so extravagant, complicated, and time consuming to prepare, that I would not include them in my healthy meal plan. My cooking methods are simple, and so are my shopping methods.

Part of my nutrition system revolves around a core group of foods. It makes shopping, preparing, storing, and creating tasty meals surprisingly easy by combining a group of ingredients compatible with many foods to create a variety of dishes. There are no long recipes with 15 steps to follow before your meal is ready. I won't follow complicated instructions for preparing my meals, and I don't expect others to do so either.

I'm often asked if I get tired or bored following the same basic list of meals week after week. My response is always the same—"no." Actually, my diet is more varied than most. Think about your food intake over a typical three-day period during the week. With the exception of dinner, most people basically eat the same foods every day. We don't require nearly the variety of food items or meals we think we do.

> Dietary habits are predominantly the key to becoming lean and reducing body fat. You cannot simply exercise your way to losing a significant amount of body fat and becoming very lean. There's a saying in the fitness industry that says "you cannot out-train a poor diet."

In the Nutrition Chapter of Part Two of this book, we will discuss the food preparation process extensively.

THE MASTER GROCERY LIST

The **Master Grocery List** (MGL) is a food shopping guide designed for use when going to the supermarket. Using the MGL, which you can find in Appendix A, you can mix and match various foods into meals that are extremely healthy and helpful in creating a lean body. You don't have to think about whether the meal you prepared is hurting your fat loss efforts, because every item on the list was carefully chosen. Each time I shop at the supermarket, I use my same list. These food items are what I eat every day.

Counting calories isn't fun. But if you create meals based off the MGL, you'll find that the need to count calories is significantly reduced as long as you don't over-consume oils, nuts, or fatty red meat.

An easy way to understand how to use the MGL in combination with a daily food log sheet is to replace any of the protein items with another type of protein in similar quantity. For example, you could replace the salmon at dinner with a steak, or the grilled chicken breast at lunch with a ground beef patty. I personally make the berry protein shake and the large mixed-green salad staple items in my diet. In other words, I eat these items every day, only changing the variety of vegetables that make up the salad and which source of protein I eat at each meal. Since quantities stay the same, it's very easy to design meals using this method. Keep in mind that the suggested total number of calories and macronutrient breakdown is considered quite aggressive in terms of preserving lean muscle while losing body fat.

I've created a 7-day example diet for you to follow (you can find this in Appendix B), which—in conjunction with the workout routines suggested in the Workout chapter of Part Two of this book—is guaranteed to dramatically help you get fit, strong, and lean. You will also become more energetic and start to experience the health benefits of eating foods that your body desires rather than the toxic chemicals that make up processed foods.

If you dine out often, this type of meal preparation lifestyle will create an enormous change that you may find challenging at first, but is ultimately rewarding. Remember, don't get caught up in the minutiae. Instead, focus on how great you'll look and feel each day you practice these life-changing habits.

Action Steps: Principle 6

Goal: Prepare the majority of your meals in advance with healthy foods using the Master Grocery List (see Appendix A).

Take action with Principle 6 starting now. This principle alone will contribute a huge percentage to your success in reducing body fat and getting lean. The recommendations here are the closest thing to "magic" that exists for losing body fat and feeling strong and healthy. Even if you do nothing else, you'll experience dramatic results in a matter of weeks simply by following this principle alone.

Principle 7:
Processed Foods Are Addictive – Like Drugs!

Remove all processed foods from your kitchen to stop the chemical addiction that occurs from eating mood-enhancing foods. For many people, even cheat meals can be dangerous.

PROCESSED FOODS AND THE OBESITY EPIDEMIC

Processed foods are the arch-enemy of health. The damage that processed foods inflict on society, in my opinion, is more harmful than all drugs and alcohol combined.

> The science on food addiction has now established that highly palatable foods (low-nutrient, high-calorie, very sweet, salty, and fatty foods—those that make up the majority of the American diet) produce the exact same biochemical effects in the brain that are characteristic of *substance abuse.*

The truth is, food addiction is worse than substance abuse because it's socially acceptable—and the foods are readily available, cheap, and in your face everywhere you look. Their consumption is promoted by grandmothers, school teachers, clergy, and even medical professionals; therefore, junk food becomes the drug of choice for many of us.

If we consider that almost two-thirds of the U.S. population is obese, and that most chronic illnesses are lifestyle-related, we can see the cost implications to the healthcare system. The cost of caring for patients with chronic illnesses is staggering because there are *no cures* for lifestyle diseases.

Long-term neglect of people's health results in management of illnesses that require years of consuming pharmaceutical drugs to manage. Epidemiologists have been predicting that the obesity epidemic is more of a threat to the U.S. economy than anything in history. Does that scare you? It should.

MOOD FOODS: THE SEROTONIN RUSH

Processed foods are filled with, for the most part, what we call empty calories— foods devoid of valuable nutrients, yet packed with calories. To depend on your willpower to refrain from consuming addictive processed foods is a fool's game.

Distinct physiological responses take place when we consume processed foods. The most important responses are neurological and result in the release of substances from the brain called **neurotransmitters**. The two most important substances associated with food addiction are **serotonin** and **dopamine**. They are often referred to as the "feel good" chemicals because of the feelings of euphoria we get from eating "mood foods."

> Similar to drugs, the addictive properties of processed foods cause you to eat more and more.

It becomes almost impossible, for example, to eat only a couple chips or one piece of chocolate fudge. Once the taste receptors are stimulated in the mouth, a strong signal is sent to the brain that causes the release of one of the neurotransmitters which increases your mood. That makes you feel good, and happy, and you continue diving into the bag for more.

STAY AWAY FROM FOOD WITH LABELS

Reading food labels is the best way we can determine the amount of processing a food has undergone. The general rule for choosing healthy food is to stay away from foods that are packaged and have complicated labeling. It's not always possible to purchase every food product without a label, but it should be a goal.

The produce sections of supermarkets do not have food labels on the fresh food items; an apple is an apple, and an eggplant is an eggplant. The majority of your diet should consist of this core group of fresh fruits and vegetables that are used to create salads and protein berry shakes similar to what I recommend in my meal preparation system.

Your next best supermarket sections are the fish and meat sections. Animal protein products also have minimal packaging and labeling because the meat is butchered and wrapped for consumers. The best way to avoid extra processing is to find a local butcher with access to quality products from 100% grass-fed animals, rather than the more commonly grain-fed animals. Eating the meat of grass-fed animals instantly increases your intake of omega-3 and omega-6 fatty acids. Animals that graze on grass have much higher levels of these vital fatty acids in their tissues than grain-fed animals. Your heart health is at stake! Choosing grass-fed over grain-fed meat can have a significant impact on your health over time.

Xenoestrogens

Eating the meat of grass-fed animals also reduces the quantity of xenoestrogens consumed. **Xenoestrogens** are estrogen-like hormone compounds that imitate estrogen, and are implicated in the creation of many undesirable conditions and serious diseases. Meat products and processed foods are the most noteworthy foods containing significant amounts of these compounds. One of the most common preservatives in processed foods that behave like a xenoestrogen is **butylated hydroxyanisole** (BHA).

Estrogen's effect on body fat levels in females is particularly interesting. Excess estrogen consumption, either through food or pharmaceutical medications, significantly hinders a woman's effort to reduce body fat—especially around the belly, hips, and thighs. For this reason alone, females should limit food sources that contain xenoestrogens.

Follow the money and you will understand why there are no paid advertisements for food products like broccoli, tomatoes, apples, spinach, cabbage, or any of the other powerful, antioxidant-containing foods that protect us against a myriad of illnesses.

> Think about it: have you ever known anyone who was obese from eating too many fresh vegetables?

It's imperative to feed children high-quality, nutrient-dense foods starting at early childhood. Large food manufacturers rely on the addictiveness of their processed foods for consistent sales, and they begin by marketing to children so the process can start at an impressionable age and continue throughout adulthood. Once children are addicted to processed foods, parents hardly stand a chance at changing their taste buds toward healthy foods.

If you've been addicted to processed foods, you *can* change that now. Without giving up the majority of processed foods, it will be significantly more difficult for you to be truly healthy, lean, fit, energetic, strong, and muscular. There's no way around it.

FOOD IS FUEL

Consciously consider how your body perceives food as fuel: you're providing it with either clean, efficient, high-grade, and energy-boosting fuel molecules, or dirty, inefficient, low-grade, and energy-zapping molecules. The organs and cells of your body provide positive feedback by demonstrating how the body functions at a higher level, and with more energy. Understanding that each cell of the human body requires high-quality nutrients for optimal functioning should inspire you to make more intelligent decisions with nutrition.

Controlling cravings

Making healthy decisions means being aware of how we often mindlessly shovel food into our mouths with no thought about its effects. We are bombarded by stimuli every moment of the day with work, cell phones, TV, music, and computers—so even when we sit down to eat a meal, we aren't mindful of what we put into our bodies.

Eating is a ritual—everyone does it. And the concept of mindfulness is not well promoted in our culture. Who has time to think about a meal when they have five minutes to get to the next activity? But society suffers deep, negative consequences from failing to adopt a healthy philosophy about the food-body connection.

Staying away from processed foods doesn't mean we will always be able to control food cravings—no one is exempt to that, even me. Over the years, I've discovered five of the best tricks and strategies to deal successfully with cravings:

1) Stop associating food with pleasure. Food is simply fuel for our body to experience premium health.
2) Keep addictive foods out of your home.
3) Replace your old habit with a new one. Are you tempted by a donut shop that you drive by on your way to work each day? Change your route.
4) Have a couple healthy replacement meals or desserts prepared that satisfy your cravings.
5) Give your cheat meal, special occasion, or holiday leftovers away—or throw them out. You don't want to feel deprived of what's sitting in your fridge. Remember, your body is not a garbage disposal!

Be kind to yourself. Have respect for your body. *Don't* pollute it with unhealthy, disease-promoting foods.

CHEAT MEALS, OR CHEAT DAYS?

Cheat meals and cheat days are popular among the most widely advertised weight loss programs because they give people "permission" to relax their willpower for a short period and eat foods they crave. In most cases, cheat meals consist of processed foods that are void of nutrition.

For example, you may cheat with pizza, or a large pasta dinner with garlic bread. Usually people prefer cheat meals that consist primarily of simple carbohydrates such as breads, pasta, and other flour-containing products. Ostensibly, a person feels less deprived and can stick to an appropriate nutrition program longer when cheat meals are permitted.

A word of caution regarding cheat meals: some people aren't able to control permitting them because it sets off a cascade of events that result in binging. It's no different than allowing a drug addict to consume a chemical they are addicted to—it ends up feeding the addiction and results in more damage than it's worth. Only you know your behavior when it comes to allowing yourself to eat outside of a healthy program. If you're someone that absolutely can't stop once you get a taste of chocolate, then maybe it's not a good idea to experiment with a cheat meal.

Cheat meals versus Cheat days

A cheat *meal* is exactly what it implies; it is one meal in which you choose to eat foods not normally permitted or consumed in your daily food program. The foods consumed can be whatever you choose, including desserts or appetizers, but are strictly limited to that specific meal and don't continue past meal time. A cheat *day* implies an entire day of consuming cheat meals.

I'm a believer of having an occasional cheat meal, but not a cheat day. Here's a good rule of thumb: feel free to choose the foods you want to consume for your cheat meal, but only for *that* sitting period. If you consume them in your house, make sure the leftover food is discarded. While many popular diet programs allow for full cheat days instead of just one cheat meal, I believe they do more harm than they're worth.

Here's why.

Consider that a person normally consumes about 2,000 calories per day to maintain a steady weight and body fat percentage. On the cheat day, they consume about 6,000 calories – three times normal consumption. (This sounds like a lot of food, but whenever you consume restaurant food heavy in simple carbohydrates and fat, as well as desserts, it's not difficult to consume 6,000 calories.) The extra 4,000 calories is more than enough to add one pound of body fat to your body. If one cheat day per week were to be included in your plan, you would gain about four pounds in a month, completely negating your efforts at keeping body fat under control.

A much better approach is to allow a cheat meal once per week. Whether it's a Saturday evening dinner or a Saturday morning brunch, you can enjoy the meal without concern for the damage to your daily efforts toward healthy eating.

Clear your home of *any* food that sends you into a binge. It's much too easy to grab "mood food" during weak moments if the food is within easy reach. Simply put, if it's not there, you can't eat it.

Action Steps: Principle 7

Goal: *Remove every processed food item from your home.*

Grab a garbage bag and fill it up! Throw away or donate *all* of your processed foods. Once your kitchen is free and clear of these items, take the MGL and go shopping. Remember, food is fuel—not a drug to be consumed after a stressful day at work. Begin looking at your body like a finely-tuned race car that needs high-grade fuel for optimal functioning. Weaning yourself off processed foods is the most challenging habit to change, but it's by far the most important—both for your health and for changing body composition to reduce fat. You must make the change. There's no way around it.

Principle 8:
There is No Magic Pill—Knowledge is Power

Stop looking for the magic pill—the "something for nothing" mentality. Understand that anything worth having requires hard work and dedication. If this wasn't the case, everyone would have it and it wouldn't be a desirable, sought-after achievement.

DON'T FALL VICTIM TO DELUSIONAL THINKING

There will never be a cure-all remedy that addresses a multi-factorial problem like obesity. The ability to consume excess food or calories without the consequences of storing fat and development of obesity would essentially mean the physiology of the human body would be circumvented. Regardless of that fact, pharmaceutical companies will continue to market the idea of a cure-all remedy simply because of the potential blockbuster profits involved.

The sooner you wipe this false notion from your brain, the sooner you'll realize the truth about what's required to transform your body and be on your way to a healthy lifestyle. I liken this analogy to that of the laws that govern nature and the universe. Certain processes can't be changed with respect to the human body. Although the idea of a cure-all remedy makes for great media headlines, nothing will become of it.

THE MAGIC IS IN POWERFUL INFORMATION

There is no magic pill in existence, and there won't likely ever be one. But an indispensable blueprint *does* exist that spells out exactly how to develop a lean, fit, and healthy body. This blueprint is the information I've developed with my program. Achieving success isn't easy, but I promise you my strategies for achieving a lean, fit, and healthy body are the most effective methods you can find, and are the same strategies I personally use every day.

I'm a scientist by trade, so I completely understand when people say they want scientific proof on a specific topic. However, I disagree with this request since you can find a credible reference for both sides of an argument. I've determined that using the scientific method to find "truth" is a futile effort—at least when it pertains to building muscle and losing fat. There are far too many conflicts of interests and biases that exist in the name of money. Behind every research article is someone with an agenda.

My recommendation to people demanding credible, research-backed information on every topic in the fitness world is to find a unbiased professional (with a following of other bias-free health professionals) that you trust, and who doesn't carry any biases or endorsements on products or supplements. Find someone whose goals align with your own; who practices the same message that he or she preaches, and remains consistent and steadfast in his or her opinions.

Success breeds success. Once you begin experiencing results, you'll become increasingly inspired by your own progress. You will begin to realize your potential to be your best. My goal is for you to achieve your best body.

Action Steps: Principle 8

Goal: Subscribe and follow the HoffmanFit blog for helpful articles on workout and fat loss tips.

If you're willing to stay on track and diligently follow my system, you're going to experience great results. As the saying goes, "you can lead a horse to water, but you can't make him drink." I'm providing the blueprint and precise steps, but ultimately *you* are responsible for putting those steps into action to form new habits that become part of your lifestyle. Stop buying into deceptive, quick-fix programs for gaining muscle and losing body fat. You're already on the right track.

Principle 9:
Get Organized

Organization increases your chances of success by saving you time—the most common reason for failing to continue a program. Organize your surroundings so you can cut the time it takes to prepare meals.

What does being organized have to do with getting lean and muscular? A lot more than you may think.

I don't know about you, but I'm much more likely to stick to a program or not be distracted when my immediate surroundings and living quarters are well organized. *HoffmanFit* is not only about transforming your body and becoming healthy, but also about being organized and efficient in a time-starved society.

We're all given the same amount of hours in a day. It's how we handle those hours which determines to a great degree what we get out of life. If we choose to squander our time performing activities using inefficient methods, we don't get much completed in a day's time.

You have probably heard the quote, "If you want something done, ask a busy person to do it." Why? Busy people are highly organized. They get things accomplished. Organization allows you to operate at full capacity, achieving the highest productivity out of life.

If you complain about not having enough time, I urge you to organize your surroundings at work and home for a dramatic improvement in your quality of life.

Some advantages of organization:

1) Reduce stress and create a sense of peace and tranquility
2) Improve quality of sleep
3) Increase feelings of control over life

4) Reduce uncertainty
5) Streamline daily processes without having to think about them
6) Feel empowered, knowing you're getting the most out of life
7) Get respect from others who notice your intelligent solutions
8) Increase self-esteem and overall satisfaction

The primary areas of focus on organizing for our purposes are food, meal preparation, and workouts.

> We are creating a systematic approach that automates the process of meal production so you can consistently eat healthy and stay lean.

FOOD ORGANIZATION

Having the MGL on hand for grocery shopping is a great start to becoming organized; by keeping the list in a place in your kitchen where you can easily mark the items you need each week, you'll always have the foods needed to prepare your meals on hand.

Create a system in your kitchen for each group of foods so you aren't confused each time you go to grab an item. Start by organizing your refrigerator. I use each shelf in my fridge for different food groups. On one shelf I'll place all my prepped lean proteins like chicken breast, hard-boiled eggs, and turkey burgers, while on another shelf I place my cut-up fresh fruits like apples and papaya. In the produce drawer, create space for your cleaned and chopped broccoli, cabbage, cauliflower, or any other vegetable that can be cleaned and placed in containers. This part of organization should be done on one of your food preparation sessions.

WORKOUT ORGANIZATION

When you're ready to implement Principle 9, you will have already decided on the amount of time you will commit each week to training, and chosen either the 4-day or 6-day workout routine. You'll know exactly what exercise you will do and how many sets and reps for each set to perform. So at this point, I highly recommend using an exercise log sheet that you can use to record your workout progress. It's important to see on paper the number of days you follow through with your workouts each week rather than trying to use your memory to recall.

Being accountable and taking responsibility will help you adhere to the program. Maintain a workout-specific calendar that you use each day only to indicate which body parts you are working so you know your focus long before the session begins. Too many people aimlessly enter the gym with no plan of action or focus because they don't know what they're working that day.

> Plan your workout schedule for a month at a time and take into account any days you will travel or have other interruptions that must be dealt with. Knowing ahead of time helps you properly plan and prepare.

In an already chaotic world, you can at least exert control over your immediate surroundings. Next to living a healthy lifestyle, being organized greatly increases the quality of our lives. By implementing the planning strategies I've provided, you'll be rewarded with the advantages of organization.

Action Steps: Principle 9

Goal: Re-organize your fridge and your kitchen with optimal efficiency in mind.

Kitchen organization is one of the best ways to properly apply the time-saving strategies of my system. Clear out everything—like dishes, pots and pans from the kitchen cupboards, and food from the pantry and refrigerator. Get rid of any food items that shouldn't be in the house like we discussed earlier. Next, create a system where all the pots and pans are systematically organized according to the location near your oven and stovetop. Reorganize the fridge based on the different food groups. Depending on the type of equipment you already own, you may have to purchase various items to properly prepare and store your food. Remember, you don't need any special equipment. My system is very basic in terms of requirements for food preparation.

Part Two:

Putting the 9 Principles in Action

The first half of this book outlined the 9 Principles important for achieving a lean & defined body. Although we discussed the basics of each principle, the rest of this book is dedicated to discussing how you can use those principles and turn them into action.

If you're interested in making a body transformation using the system I use with my clients, you can be a part of my next 12-Week Body Transformation Coaching Program.

Maybe the information in this book is overwhelming for you to start implementing your new fitness lifestyle and you could use help. My transformation system is a one-of-a-kind program that helps people just like you who may have minimal knowledge about how to cohesively put all this information together.

You can find out more details about my program by visiting my website to see if you want to make a life-changing decision to get in the best shape of your life: http://www.hoffmanfit.com

Workouts & Training

Ask yourself two questions: (1) what do you want to accomplish by working out and eating healthy, and (2) how much time are you willing to dedicate to working toward that goal? Here is a list of the most common goals people tell me they'd like to achieve from working out and eating healthy:

1) To look good in all clothes, whether it is in jeans or dress clothes
2) To look good in a swimsuit and various sports attire
3) To increase strength and stamina
4) To increase energy levels
5) To increase self-confidence and self-esteem
6) To improve overall health and prevent lifestyle-related diseases from occurring so early in life
7) To improve sleep and recovery habits
8) To improve sex life and the ability to attract a mate

The primary goal of this book is to teach you how to develop a lean, muscular, and defined body; the remaining goals listed above go hand-in-hand with the system I've developed.

COMPOUND AND MULTI-JOINT EXERCISES

There's no magic in doing one exercise versus another—no "spot reducing" like many people desperately want to believe. Instead, there is a group of exercises that are excellent at producing results due to how they stimulate the largest numbers of muscle fibers. These are what we referred to earlier as **compound** or **multi-joint exercises**.

For each muscle group in the body, there are several exercises that ultimately produce the same results whether you're looking to get fit and strong or to gain and shape muscle with bodybuilding. Don't be deceived into thinking certain exercises produce a major difference in body shape or conditioning versus others. To a large degree, your muscles develop according to a pre-determined shape that is encoded within your DNA. However, hard work and dedication can certainly override genetics. When I refer to genetics, I'm talking about features like length of the muscle and other characteristics that can't be altered regardless of how hard you work. For example, you can't elongate your muscles by doing Pilates, regardless of what Pilates experts say.

CHOOSING YOUR WORKOUT SPACE

Home-Based Workouts

As our lives become busier every year, the thought of a home gym can be enticing. Here are some reasons why people choose to work out at home instead of the gym:

- Home workouts save time traveling to and from the gym
- Gyms can be intimidating and/or lack privacy
- There's no waiting in line for equipment during peak gym hours
- If there are children in the home, there is no need for child care during the workout session

While some are able to enjoy these benefits, it's important to understand that there are several drawbacks and obstacles to setting up a home fitness studio. For example, while you might save time working out at home versus driving to the gym and potentially waiting for equipment, it doesn't matter in the end if you don't *actually* work out. My observation (over three decades of experience) is that the success rate of those who work out at home is low. A quick search on Craigslist could convince anyone of this. There are countless ads for new or like new fitness equipment that "just sits in our rec room; we hardly ever use it."

Consider the following regarding home gyms:

- **Space** – In order to have a successful home gym, you must have a large open area—or even a dedicated room—for workout space. You may need to re-organize or get rid of some furniture to give you enough room for a proper workout area.

- **Money** – A home gym can be a major investment. Quality equipment is the only equipment worth investing in, and it can become very expensive.

- **Distractions** – The home can be a very distracting place. Phone calls, text messages, television, neighbors, or children are examples of what could totally sabotage your workout. At the gym, it is easier to focus and separate yourself from such distractions.

- **Environment** – Your home is designed by you to be your place of comfort; it's your place to eat, sleep, and live. That level of comfort often makes it difficult to get motivated and work up a sweat in that space.

Despite these obstacles, many people *are* able to make home gyms work for them, and are disciplined enough to achieve real results. The ability to make home gyms work successfully might depend on your personality and how in tune you are with your own habits in certain environments.

If you're the type of person who feeds off the energy of others, the home gym environment may leave you feeling lazy or uninspired as a workout area. If you're the type of person who gains energy from solitude, your workout focus might be best in the home gym environment.

In my experience, performing workouts in a home gym doesn't work for many individuals. I'll admit that I'm biased toward training in a gym. On two different occasions I've put together a home gym. In my experience, my workouts weren't nearly as effective as they were at a commercial facility. The potential for a great workout was there, but the motivation wasn't. Read over the list of concerns above once more. If you are an exception and can work out from home with minimal equipment, go for it! You can certainly save some valuable time. Over the years, I've trained some working professionals who prefer to work out from home because of time demands. They've been very successful at following a program and achieving great results.

***

If you decide to go with the home-based gym route, here are some helpful tips and guidelines for setting it up.

Size of workout area

Based on my equipment recommendations, you should need approximately 100 square feet. I don't recommend spending the money on bulky machines and treadmills that take up a lot of space.

Basic equipment needed

The following equipment consists of what I consider the bare minimum necessary in order to get results comparable to what you could get at a gym. Although you can do body-weight exercises, they won't produce the same results as free weights. If you're going to engage in a workout routine, you should strive to get the most results from your efforts. There are too many exercises that you won't be able to perform without dumbbells or barbells.

Adjustable weight bench

Estimated cost: $175-$250

Adjustable benches allow you to perform movements flat on your back and at an incline. Since they give you more options for different exercises and make good use of space, it's worth spending a little more for this feature. You can purchase a weight bench at any major sporting goods or online store. There's no need to spend the money for a commercial-quality bench since you'll only be using it in your home.

Set of adjustable dumbbells

Estimated cost: $175 for women, $275 for men

There are many different types of dumbbells, and there are advantages and disadvantages to each kind. Since space is a consideration for most, I recommend the Power Block adjustable dumbbells because one set replaces 10 individual pairs of dumbbells. Improvements over the years have made them comfortable to use. In a matter of seconds, you can change the weight of the dumbbell without having to remove standard weights. Additionally, they take up very little space so you don't have many sets of weights spread all over your workout area.

If you aren't able to go with this option, you can purchase individual, fixed-iron dumbbells. The problem with this style of dumbbell is you'll need many different weights for doing various exercises. As your strength increases, you'll need heavier weights after just a couple months. You won't be able to train effectively if you don't have the proper weight required to progressively overload your muscles.

Barbell or EZ-curl bar with collars:

Estimated cost: $75-$150

Although your home gym will include a full set of dumbbells, it is well worth the extra money to add a barbell to the equipment list due to its versatility and the strength and muscle gains it can produce.

For beginners, I suggest using a straight barbell because it will help you develop balance and coordination more than the shorter E-Z curl barbell. The most noteworthy advantage of the E-Z curl bar is the tension it removes from the wrist when performing bicep curls or skull crushers to work your triceps.

You will also need to purchase some plate weights to use with the bar. The standard seven-foot Olympic bar weighs 45 pounds, which isn't heavy enough for males to perform many exercises—even beginners. You can start by purchasing a couple of 5- and 10-pound plates, then move up to 25-pound plates as your strength progresses. Go with a straight barbell because it will teach you to develop balance and coordination more than the shorter E-Z curl barbell.

In order to hold the plates in place on the barbell, you'll need collars. There are many different styles of collars, but I prefer the quick-lock type that easily slides on and off for quicker changing of weights. Clip-style collars are also available, but they sometimes slide off the ends and create a dangerous situation.

Pull-up bar:

Estimated cost: $30 - $80

A home gym isn't complete without a pull-up bar. Most manufacturer models fit all doorways and don't require any installation or drilling of holes for use. Note: there are many people that aren't physically able to perform one complete pull-up. By using a chair for assistance you can gradually increase your strength until you can perform on your own.

After conducting some research on the different pull-up bars available, I've narrowed it down to two great manufacturers: The Iron Gym Total Upper Body Workout Bar or Beach Body's Pro-grade chin-up bar for P90X.

Swiss ball (stability ball)

Estimated cost: $30

Purchase a Swiss ball according to your height. The sizes range between 45-75 cm and can be purchased at any sporting goods store. You'll need a stability ball for almost every workout to work out your abdominals and other core muscles.

Exercise mat

Estimated cost: $35

An exercise mat is needed for stretching before every workout and for doing several exercises. The mat creates padding and cushions your back, allowing for a more comfortable stretching experience versus lying on a hard floor. Find one that can fold or roll up to place in a closet.

Total Cost

Now that we've determined the equipment needed for a home gym, let's take a look at the total costs involved.

- Adjustable workout bench: $175-250
- Adjustable dumbbell set: $175-275
- Barbell or E-Z curl bar with plate weights: $75-150
- Pull-up bar: $30-$80
- Swiss ball/Stability ball: $30
- Exercise mat: $30

Total cost of equipment: $515 – $815

Create a Home Gym Environment for Success

Distractions can easily sabotage your home workout goals. A great solution is to schedule your workouts just like any other appointment on your calendar. Choose a time that doesn't conflict with other responsibilities and *follow through* with the plan. If you honor this time commitment, your home gym will prove to be a success.
Since motivation, or the lack thereof, is the number one issue in being consistent with productive home workouts, I've created a list of suggestions of things you can do in order to stay motivated:

- Set up your iPod or other device to play music that inspires you.
- Use a fan, or open windows or doors that will create movement of air for better ventilation.
- Get a journal and start tracking your workouts so that you see your progress. Record which body parts you train, weights used, number of sets, and repetitions performed. You'll be much more cognizant about what you're doing if you see everything on paper.
- Put away your phone. The number one habit I see at the gym is people playing with their cell phones. Get your music prepared before your workout and don't play around with your phone until you've completed your entire workout.

Making a Decision

Are you still unsure of which route to take when considering a gym membership versus setting up a home gym? Use the question guides I've provided below to help you decide.

Consider a commercial gym or health club if you fit the following profile:

1) The gym is located close and is convenient to use.

2) You enjoy the surroundings of a gym and the energy of other people.

3) You will be distracted and not likely to work out from home.

Consider a home gym if you fit the following:

1) You're self-disciplined and motivated to work out from home

2) You won't be easily distracted by family members, phone calls or TV.

3) You have the space and will invest in the minimal equipment required.

4) Gym workouts are too time-consuming for your schedule, and location is not convenient.

5) Completing workouts in 30 minutes is the only way you'll consistently workout.

FINDING THE RIGHT GYM

Not a fan of fitness clubs? I get it. I've done a lot of "club hopping" in the past because I didn't like the feel of certain fitness centers. But at the end of the day, you and I have goals to achieve, and personal preferences can't get in the way. Here are the important questions:

- Is the gym or fitness center I'm considering conveniently located to your home or work?
- Do they have a decent set of dumbbells so you can perform the workout necessary to reach your goals?

If the answer to both questions is yes, forget the other details.

Regarding gym memberships, note this: *don't* get fooled into signing a long-term contract. Nearly every gym and fitness center offers a month-to-month system, even if all a representative tries to discuss with you is a long-term commitment. With a month-by-month contract, you may be charged for one month in advance, but you can opt out at any time. And always tell them you don't want to pay any start-up fees. In fact, if they don't offer it up front, you should request a one- or two-week free pass to test the club out beforehand. They want you as a member, so you're entitled to ask for reasonable accommodations.

CHOOSING A WORKOUT ROUTINE

Now it's time to decide which workout routine will fit with your schedule and goals.
The more time you invest in training, the more results you're going to get.

The 12-minute, three-times-a-week workouts you read about online (which "produce amazing results!") are a lie. Another lie is the concern about over-training that a lot of gimmicky programs warn you about. It's nothing but a marketing ploy—if I get amazing results and don't have to work out as often, I should buy in to it, right? Sounds great!

Let's get real. Meaningful changes to your body require a considerable amount of training for almost everybody. Even at my level of fitness, I still have to train at least four times per week while hitting each muscle group two times over an eight-day period in order to maintain current levels.

What does over-training a muscle mean? Over-training a muscle can occur when the same muscle group is trained more than once within a 48-hour period. This is much different than simply stating "you shouldn't work out every day." See the difference?

> You can work out every day as long as the individual muscle groups have two full days of rest before they are trained again.

The split routine workout schedule I've created has been carefully crafted to include the necessary two days of rest between muscle groups. Take a look at the following schedules and decide which one you think will work best for your schedule and lifestyle. Each workout takes less than 45 minutes to complete, or around 30 minutes if you work out from home. Regardless of workout location, the exercises listed in the schedule are similar (some alternative exercises are provided due to the equipment limitations of a home gym), and will produce similar results.

4-day vs. 6-day routines

The primary difference in the 4-day routine versus the 6-day routine is that the 6-day workout routine is split into what is termed a **push/pull/legs split routine**. This split is a weight training schedule that revolves around splitting the body into 3 groups: upper body pushing muscles, upper body pulling muscles, and legs. Each group is then trained separately on its own workout day as indicated in the charts below. This style of split routine is one of the most effective training routines for strengthening and shaping each muscle of your body. It places an emphasis on each muscle group versus only performing movements that don't target individual muscles as well. The push/pull/legs split routine also allows you to add more volume to your workouts because you only train two or three muscle groups per session instead of working out the entire upper body in a single workout.

Factors to consider for choosing between the 4-day vs. 6-day workout routines

Start with a **4-day routine** if you fit the following profile:

1) You are a novice to weight training

2) You cannot devote more than four sessions of training per week

3) You are OK with achieving minimal results and aren't looking for a serious body transformation

Start with a **6-day routine** if you fit the following profile:

1) You already have experience lifting free weights (dumbbells, barbells, cable machines)

2) You're willing to devote the time for six workout sessions per week

3) You're dedicated to achieving serious results and are willing to do what is required

4) You want to develop more shape and definition to your body

WORKING THROUGH INITIAL SORENESS

Expect to experience some muscle soreness in the first 10 days of working out. This is called **delayed onset muscle soreness,** or DOMS as it's referred to in exercise physiology. This is normal, and there's nothing you can do to eliminate it. You'll hear a hundred different remedies for reducing the soreness such as getting a massage or winding down in a whirlpool, but nothing has been proven to reduce the soreness.

The soreness is thought to be a result of the micro-trauma caused to the individual muscle fibers being exercised, although the exact cause of soreness is not known. The micro-trauma also increases your metabolism since the body utilizes extra calories as the energy required to repair the damaged muscle fibers.

Once your body becomes accustomed to a few workouts, the soreness will subside until you increase intensity. Don't worry, soreness isn't a bad thing; it's like a wake-up call to your muscles—you know that something good is happening.

Workouts & Training for the 40+ population: Boomer-itis

Society has brainwashed people aged 40 and up into thinking that, as we age each year, we automatically start losing the physical capabilities of doing certain things concerning workouts or other areas of life. It's like we're screwed from the start of middle age. This is a topic I'm very passionate about because it involves people from my generation (or somewhere close to this age). Next to the myth that women bulk up from lifting heavy weights, the second-biggest myth is that middle-aged people need to take care not to lift heavy weights because they will get hurt or injured.

It's time to put this myth to rest.

The truth is the opposite: if you don't strengthen your body with weight training, you may face the awful condition of sarcopenia. **Sarcopenia**[1] is the degenerative loss of skeletal muscle mass (0.5-1% loss per year after the age of 25), quality, and strength associated with aging. Although sarcopenia is predominantly seen in those that are inactive, it also occurs to a lesser degree in those that are active. This suggests there are other factors involved in sarcopenia besides inactivity.

Researchers believe the following factors also play a role in sarcopenia:

- A reduction in the body's ability to synthesize protein
- Decrease in hormones such as GH, testosterone and insulin-like growth factor
- Age-related reduction in nerve cells that send signals from the brain to muscles to initiate movement
- Insufficient intake of calories and protein to maintain muscle mass[2]

The only treatment to prevent sarcopenia is exercise—specifically resistance or strength training with free weights.

Surprised?

---

[1] Wikipedia definition: http://en.wikipedia.org/wiki/Sarcopenia
[2] WebMD definition: http://www.webmd.com/healthy-aging/sarcopenia-with-aging

We've been trained by the false mindset that says there should be "special programs," "special diets," and "special" everything since you're older, and that's the way it is. It's the default response to "why is this aching?" "Because you're getting older!" I like to refer to the condition of every middle-aged person that has aches and pains as "boomer-itis" instead of tendonitis. And it's the biggest lie you've ever been told. You can't change your chronological age, but you *can* determine your mental age. When we "think like an old person," our actions tend to follow suit. Think younger.

I achieved the best physical condition of my life at 54 years old. My body has been conditioned to its peak, and my blood tests indicate the body of a man in his 20s biologically. The exercise routines (which are the same ones I did at 20 years old) and nutritional habits I follow have caused a powerful anti-aging effect. Don't get caught up thinking that I am "the exception," and this won't work for you. I've helped countless men and women around my age start fresh and achieve the same results as I have. It's never too late to start a health and fitness program.

Don't get me wrong, I'm not telling you to go out and start wielding weights like a mad man because your age isn't a factor. If you do that, you most certainly *will* get injured, just as I would if I didn't first condition my body and then progressively train until I got used to the weights. All I'm saying is you are *not* limited in a major way because of your age. I've worked with clients all the way up to 88 years old. I recently coached a female who does CrossFit at 60 years old and kicks butt over women in their 20s. And she's only been lifting for a few years!

INJURIES, ACHES, AND PAINS

The biggest concerns from middle-aged people are injuries, aches, and pains. While these are valid concerns, I've concluded that not working out only makes matters worse. Your body deteriorates at an accelerated rate once you reach your late 30s unless you work out to preserve your muscle mass. If people are willing to work through some of the aches and pains they initially encounter, they'll discover that many of the pains will eventually subside.

First, let me express something important—I've been training for 37 years, and I'm no stranger to injuries. I live with several serious injuries, and I've tolerated chronic pain for the past four years. I've even undergone some procedures to help ease the pain. In spite of this, I still managed to train at an extremely advanced level.

I'm completely convinced that the majority of aches and pains are used as an excuse to avoid lifting weights. There will always be exceptions to this, but I'm speaking about the majority of cases. An additional point to consider is that injuries often result from performing simple tasks like tossing a ball for your dog, or getting out of bed in the morning. Aches and pains are experienced from doing anything when you get older, but avoiding exercise only exacerbates the problem more. It's wrong and unfair to associate lifting weights to your injury in every case.

It's not just society that feeds us the lines "be careful," "don't over-exert yourself," or, "don't lift any weight" to those with physical ailments. Doctors play into it too, and provide their opinion by almost always telling the patient to abstain from any exercise.

Does anyone realize that the reason for most aches and pains is muscle atrophy and the weakening of tendons, ligaments, and associated connective tissue in the joints of the body? If everyone started engaging in some type of physical activity tomorrow, I believe half the treatments that are administered would be wiped out as a result.

There are many effective ways to train around a serious or non-serious injury. The problem is, many people like to use injury as an excuse and completely refrain from working out altogether. Unfortunately, aches and pains will only become worse as your musculature continues to atrophy and become weak. No single activity will increase vitality more, regardless of age, than exercise. By not engaging in exercise that prevents the loss of muscle tissue, you'll set yourself up for a huge array of diseases, all related in some way to the dreaded condition of sarcopenia that seldom is talked about.

WHAT MAKES YOU OLD?

Have you ever realized that (despite actual age), we "get old" primarily due to the people we spend our time with? I typically hang out with people much younger than me since I choose to surround myself with active, energetic people who share my goals of personal excellence in health and fitness. What we believe to be "normal" about our age progression and its correlating behaviors is based on our mind's unique interpretation of "normal." If what we're witnessing in the behaviors of people we hang out with is "old," that becomes our reality and we accept it as truth. We are essentially programmed from the start to think this way.

Get rid of the "I'm getting old" mindset. Society tends to picture middle-aged people with one foot in the grave and sets these ridiculous limits on what those people can physically do. Is that what you want for yourself? Would you settle for that? I hope not.

As I mentioned, I tend to surround myself with younger, energetic people; often these friends are at least 15 years younger than me. I first realized how different my surroundings were at the last high school reunion I attended (more than a decade ago). The people I saw were the people I grew up with, attended school with, played sports with, and then didn't see for over 25 years. I couldn't even recognize the majority of them without looking at their name tags. What they did during the years that followed high school versus what I did resulted in an astounding physical difference.

> What you do to your body determines how you age both externally and internally.

Even at middle age you have an incredible opportunity to take control of your health during the second half of your life and start treating your body with respect. In return, you will slow down the aging process and thwart the debilitating effects that inactivity and poor nutritional habits have on every aspect of your life.

Muscle is the greatest commodity in existence, and everything you do in terms of health and fitness should revolve around gaining and preserving muscle tissue. In fact, the amount of muscle tissue a person possesses is the greatest determinant of health. These types of "biomarkers" (measured characteristics which can be used as indicators to certain states or conditions of health) are now a common analytical tool used to determine one's health, longevity, and the percentage of lean muscle mass that is considered at the top of the chart of importance to one's health.

It's absolutely amazing to coach a client and see the changes that occur to his or her body and overall health. My favorite group of individuals to train are those between their 40s and 60s. The remarkable changes and improvements that typically occur to their bodies have proved to be some of my greatest achievements with client transformations.

TESTIMONIALS

There is nothing more powerful than seeing the results for yourself. Here are some powerful testimonies from two past clients of mine.

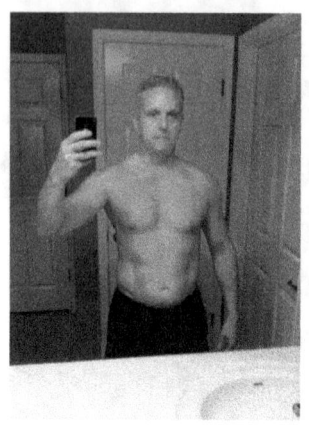 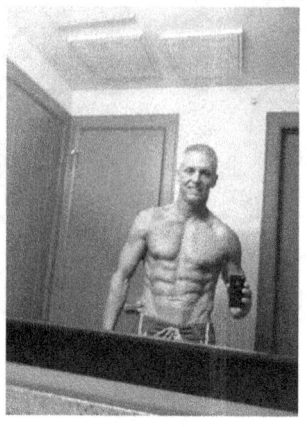

Before   **After**

I'm a 50 year retired Army Veteran. I have been fairly athletic my entire life, keeping myself in shape, and eating what I thought to be "healthy"! After 10 years of military retirement and living somewhat of a sedentary lifestyle, my body began to go into a down-hill spiral. I knew I needed to make a change, but I wasn't quite sure how to do it on my own.

I heard about Philip Hoffman through a friend and decided to visit his Facebook page "HoffmanFit." After reading several of the posts on his page, I purchased his book, The 9 Principles For a Lean and Defined Body. I couldn't put it down. When I saw the Facebook post advertising Phil's 12-week Six-Pack Ab Challenge, I emailed Phil and asked if I could take part in it. After corresponding through email, I was in the challenge! The next 12 weeks changed my life FOREVER!

I went into the challenge weighing 188lbs at 5'10" in height with a waist size of 36". Some would say that's not too bad. However, I wasn't happy with my body and as a middle-aged man, I knew it would continue to get worse! In a very short period of time, I came to trust in Phil and his credentials, and realized the true sustainability of his program. It is not a crash diet!

Philip worked very closely with each and every person in the challenge. We were educated on weight training, using proper form & technique, high-intensity training, time-under-tension, and more. We were introduced to proper nutrition, calories/macronutrient breakdown, food preparation, and given some of the best recipes that were very quick and easy to make! I followed the HoffmanFit *program to the "T". After 12 weeks, I lost over 20 lbs, my waist had gone from 36" to 30", my entire body was totally ripped, I had a ton of energy, and my confidence had skyrocketed! I am so grateful to Philip Hoffman and highly recommend the* HoffmanFit *program to anyone looking to live a healthy & sustainable lifestyle!*

Loan-Anh

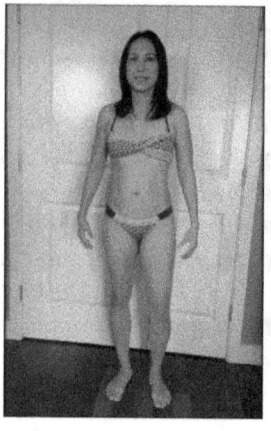 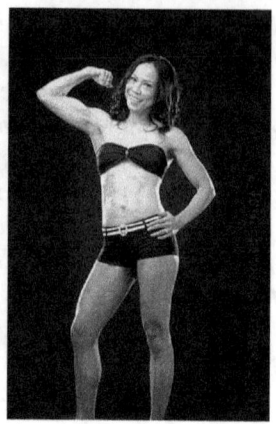

Before   **After**

"Before reading Phil's article 'Do Women Bulk-Up by lifting Heavy Weights?' I knew that I wanted my body to look something like the woman on the cover. After reading, I contacted Phil to thank him for writing such an informative article; not long after he connected back with me, I was invited to be a part of his first online abs challenge contest. When I started training, I was 125 lbs. I am 5 feet, 4 inches tall, and most people would call that an acceptable size. However, after giving birth to two children, I knew I had to lose some fat around my abdominal and glute areas. All I wanted was to look good in a bikini at the beach! With Phil's incredible support and motivation, I was able to follow his easy-to-follow plan and achieve results within 12 weeks! If you're determined enough to try the plan and make it a priority, you can get there too—and you'll never want to turn back.

The plan itself is simple—no gimmicks!—and there's no starving yourself or putting yourself on a quick cleanse, prohibitive diet, or constant workouts. If you think you're too old to try new things, whether it is with fitness, cooking, or career, you're wrong. I am in my forties, I have 2 children, a full-time job, celiac disease, and a severe dairy allergy. But this system worked for me! Don't let yourself become discouraged. You are the captain of your own ship, and at the end of the day no one is accountable for your life except you."

Me

My most recent achievements in 2013 should clearly illustrate the point that your best body ever can still be achieved at middle age. I'm extremely proud of what I've worked hard to achieve, and I plan on taking my message to the middle-aged generation throughout the world.

2013 was an amazing year for me. My workout routine and nutritional program was adjusted to help me get in the most muscular and leanest condition ever—even better than my 20s. The year started out by doing a featured cover shoot and article in Scottsdale Health Magazine, local to my city. After the magazine was released, I was bombarded with many emails from middle-aged folks asking me what I did to stay so fit, strong, and young-looking. I didn't realize how different I was in physical condition compared to people close to my age because I'm rarely around anyone my age at the gym.

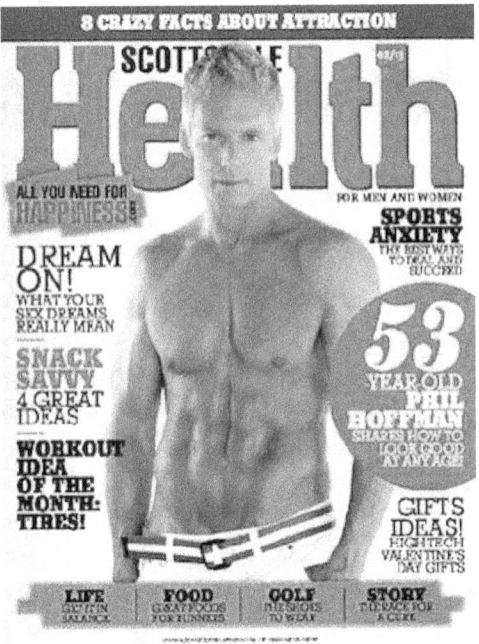

For the past four years I've scheduled photo shoots on my birthday to mark the celebration of another year of hard work of training and healthy nutritional practices. In 2013 I surpassed all previous years in terms of physical condition and body fat reduction. By further testing my program's methods and applying the knowledge I've acquired throughout my life, I was able to reach my goals despite my age

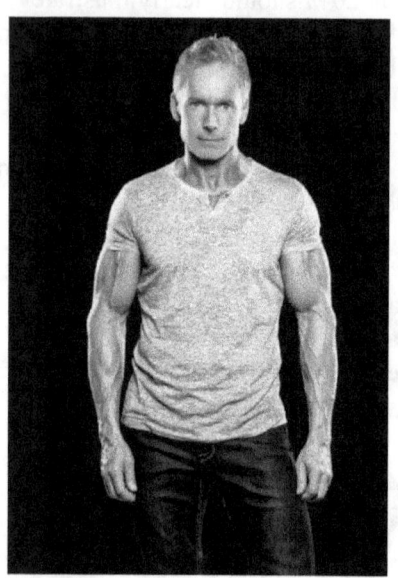 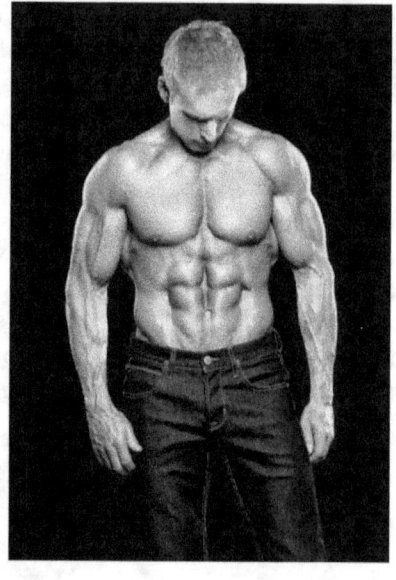

If you follow my program, I highly recommend taking photos each year to document your progress. It's a great way to stay inspired and watch your body improve even though your chronological age is increasing. *This* is how you slow the aging process.

Never think you can't get into the best condition of your life—even if you're over 50 years old. If you're truly committed, determined, and dedicated enough to achieve the goal of getting into the best shape of your life, you absolutely can!

Workout Plans

Once you choose between the 4- or 6-day routines, you're ready to follow the plan. The following workouts are separated into gym-based and home-based routines due to the differences in necessary equipment. The workouts are further divided according to beginner and intermediate levels.

WARMING UP

Regardless of where you work out, you need to warm up before jumping into your routine. The best way to warm up for strength training is to choose a light weight and perform the exact exercise you'll be performing with heavier weight. This allows for the muscles to go through the same range of motion you'll be doing and start to shift blood to that area of your body.

For example, if you're about to perform squats for quadriceps, choose a light weight that you can easily perform 20 or more repetitions with, yet only perform 15. Rest one minute and perform another set with a weight slightly heavier and perform 15 repetitions again.

Now you're ready to begin performing the number of sets indicated in your workout schedule. Do not include your warm-up sets as part of your workout for the first exercise of each body part, however. You won't need to warm up for the second exercise of each body part since what you're working is already warmed up. If you were to perform warm-up sets for each exercise you wouldn't have enough energy to properly perform the heavier sets.

Here's an example of how to include warm-up sets for leg workouts that include 3 exercises: squats, lunges and Romanian dead lifts.

1) *Warm-up set 1 for squats*: Perform squats doing 15 reps with a weight that you can perform 20 reps with.
2) *Warm-up set 2 for squats*: Perform squats doing 15 reps with a weight slightly heavier than warm-up set 1.
3) Perform your first set of squats and the remaining sets of squats according to your routine.
4) *Lunges*: No warm-up set required since your legs are already

warmed up from several sets of squats.

5) *Romanian dead lifts*: Perform one warm up before moving into your real sets. The reason you perform a warm-up set here, even though your legs are already warmed up, is because there's a significant difference in the type of exercise movement here.

6) Now perform the prescribed number of sets of Romanian dead-lifts according to the workout you're following.

*This exercise is an exception and warrants an extra warm-up set to really stretch the lower back and hamstring muscles. Ensuring sufficient blood supply is shunted to this area as well as strong neural signals from the brain in preparation for physical exertion is important in this region of the body.

Be careful not to confuse *exercises* with *sets*. They have two completely different meanings as used in this context. **Exercises** refer to a specific movement performed to work a body part. Examples are squats and lunges for legs, or pull-ups and one-arm rows for the back. **Sets** refer to the number of each exercise you perform for a given exercise. For example, you perform three sets of squats. People mistakenly say they did three exercises for squats when the correct way to state this is they did three sets of squats.

DETERMINING STARTING WEIGHT FOR EXERCISES

Determining the correct starting weight for each exercise requires some trial and error. Find a weight that challenges you to do about 10 reps. Since you generally perform 3-4 sets per exercise, the weight will feel significantly heavier after each set. Find the exact weight that challenges you, yet allows the execution of good form throughout every set.

Finding a moderate weight to use for each exercise is important because it will serve as the baseline strength point for all your sets. Females tend to be timid of weights and end up using a poundage that is too light for them; muscles are not sufficiently stimulated as a result. The myth of bulking up from lifting heavy weights is so engrained in the minds of women that appropriate weights are seldom used in workouts.

Males, on the other hand, tend to let their egos get involved and sacrifice form and technique in order to push weights that are too heavy. I can't stress enough how important proper form is for building quality

74

muscle and preventing injuries. You will stimulate muscular growth to a larger degree by using lighter weights and performing good form than by using heavier weights and performing poor form.

The starting weight you choose should allow you a range of performing 15 reps at the maximum and 8 reps at the minimum. If you're able to perform 15 reps without any level of difficulty, you need to increase the weight. If you're struggling with 8 repetitions, you need to reduce the weight. Be sure to write down your weights when you start your program or you'll never remember which weights to choose for each workout. Start by performing a set with a weight you can perform 20 reps with if you had to.

***

The following charts indicate estimated starting weights for both females and males for each exercise. They should be used as a guide to establish the weights you will use for your workouts until you get through the initial soreness period and become accustomed to the exercises.

Note that weights are based on beginner level lifters that either have no experience lifting, or have not worked out over the past year. These are only estimates, and not everyone will fall within these ranges to start. Also note that novice males are not significantly stronger that novice females. For most of the exercises, males are roughly 25% stronger than females. That's not based on any formal studies, but from what I've actually experienced while training hundreds of clients over 30 years of time.

*Dumbbells = DB, Barbell = BB

Estimated starting weight (females)

Legs:		
Name of Exercise	**Dumbbell/Barbell Weight**	**Exercise Machine**
DB Squats	10-15 lbs. (set of DBs)	
Goblet Squats	10-15 lbs. (one DB)	
Romanian deadlifts	10-15 lbs. (set of DBs)	
DB lunges	5-10 lbs. (set of DBs)	

Leg press		25-45 lb. plate (each side)
Lying leg curls		40-60 lbs.
Seated calf raises		35-45 lb. plate
One-leg calf raises	10-15 lbs. (one DB)	

Back:		
Name of Exercise	**Dumbbell/Barbell Weight**	**Exercise Machine**
Pull-ups (assisted)	Use bands to assist	Trial & error method
Wide-grip cable pull downs		40-60 lbs.
Seated cable row		30-50 lbs.
One-arm DB row	10-15 lbs. (one DB)	
Bent-over BB row	20-30 lbs. (BB)	
Deadlift	65-75 lbs. (Olympic BB)	
T-bar row		25-35 lbs.
Pull-overs w/DB	15-20 lbs. (one DB)	

Chest:		
Name of Exercise	**Dumbbell/Barbell Weight**	**Exercise Machine**
DB bench press	10-15 lbs.	
Incline DB press	10-12 lbs.	
DB flys	8-10 lbs.	
DB flys on Swiss ball	8-10 lbs.	

Shoulders:		
Name of Exercise	**Dumbbell/Barbell Weight**	**Exercise Machine**
Seated DB press	8-10 lbs.	
DB side raises	5-8 lbs.	
DB rear raises	5-8 lbs.	
Upright DB rows	8-10 lbs.	

Triceps:		
Name of Exercise	**Dumbbell/Barbell Weight**	**Exercise Machine**
Cable pressdowns		40-50 lbs.
Lying EZ bar extension (skull crushers)	20-25 lbs.(use EZ bar)	
Bench dips	Body weight only	
Behind head DB extension	10-15 lbs. (one DB)	

Biceps:		
Name of Exercise	**Dumbbell/Barbell Weight**	**Exercise Machine**
Standing barbell curl	20-25 lbs. (BB)	
Seated DB curls	10-12 lbs. (set of DBs)	

Abs:		
Name of Exercise	**Dumbbell/Barbell Weight**	**Exercise Machine**
Front & side planks	Body weight only	
Swiss ball crunches	Body weight only	
Captain chair knee raises	Body weight only	Captain's chair apparatus

*Note: when an exercise indicates DB weight it always means a set (2) of DBs unless the exercise is performed with one DB such as the goblet squat.

Estimated starting weight (Males)

Legs:		
Name of Exercise	**Dumbbell/Barbell Weight**	**Exercise Machine**
DB Squats	15-20 lbs.	
Goblet Squats	20-25 lbs.	
Romanian deadlifts	15-25 lbs.	
DB lunges	10-15 lbs.	
Leg press		35-45 lb. plates (2)
Lying leg curls		50-70 lbs.
Seated calf raises		35-45 lb. plate
One-leg calf raises	15-20 lbs.	

Back:		
Name of Exercise	**Dumbbell/Barbell Weight**	**Exercise Machine**
Pull-ups (assisted)		Trial and error method
Wide-grip pull downs		60-80 lbs.
Seated cable row		60-70 lbs.
One-arm DB row	20-25 lbs.	
Bent-over BB row	40-50 lbs.(BB)	
Deadlift	95-115 lbs.	
T-bar row		35-45 lbs.
Pull-overs w/DB	20-25 lbs.	

Chest:		
Name of Exercise	**Dumbbell/Barbell Weight**	**Exercise Machine**
DB bench press	20-30 lbs.	
Incline DB press	20-25 lbs.	
DB flys	15-20 lbs.	
DB flys on Swiss ball	12-15 lbs.	

Shoulders:		
Name of Exercise	**Dumbbell/Barbell Weight**	**Exercise Machine**
Seated DB press	12-15 lbs.	
DB side raises	10-12 lbs.	
DB rear raises	10-12 lbs.	
Upright DB rows	12-15 lbs.	

Triceps:		
Name of Exercise	**Dumbbell/Barbell Weight**	**Exercise Machine**
Cable pressdowns		60-80 lbs.
Lying EZ bar extension (skull crushers)	25-30 lbs. (use EZ bar)	
Behind the neck DB extension	20-25 lbs.	
Bench dips	Body weight only	

Biceps:		
Name of Exercise	**Dumbbell/Barbell Weight**	**Exercise Machine**
Standing BB curl	30-35 lbs. (bb)	
Seated DB curl	15-20 lbs.	

Abs:		
Name of Exercise	**Dumbbell/Barbell Weight**	**Exercise Machine**
Front & side plank	Body weight only	
Swiss ball crunches	Body weight only	
Captain's chair leg knee raises	Body weight only	Captain's chair apparatus

*Note: when an exercise indicates the DB weight, it always means a set (2) of DBs used unless the exercise is performed with one DB such as the goblet squat.

Workout Schedules

GYM-BASED WORKOUT SCHEDULES

4-day workout schedule (beginner)

Monday & Thursday: Chest, Back, Biceps and Triceps

Exercise	Sets	Reps	Rest
*DB bench press	4	8-10	*45-60 seconds
Incline DB press	4	8-10	*
Wide-grip cable pull down	3	8-10	*
Bent-over DB row	3	8-10	*
Pull-ups (assisted)	3	10-12	*
Skull crushers (E-Z bar)	3	8-10	*
Cable press downs	3	8-10	*
Standing BB curls	4	8-10	*

*DB – Dumbbell, BB – Barbell

Tuesday & Friday: Legs, Shoulders and Abdominals

Exercise	Sets	Reps	Rest
DB squats or goblet squats	3	8-10	*
Romanian deadlifts	3	8-10	*
DB lunges	3	8-10	*
Seated DB press	4	8-10	*
DB side raises	4	8-10	*

| Bicycle crossovers | 3 | 15-20 | * |
| V-ups | 3 | 20-25 | * |

6-Day Workout Schedule (intermediate)

Monday & Thursday: Chest, Triceps, Abs

*Abdominal muscles worked 3x per week

Exercise	Sets	Reps	Rest
DB bench press	4	8-10	*
Incline DB press	4	8-10	*
DB fly or cable fly	4	10-12	*
Skull crushers (E-Z bar)	4	8-10	*
Cable pressdowns	4	10-12	*
Bicycle crossovers	3	15-20	*
V-ups	3	20-25	*
Reverse crunch w/stability ball	3	15-20	*

*Abdominal muscles worked 3x per week

Tuesday & Friday: Back, Biceps

Exercise	Sets	Reps	Rest
Pull ups (assisted)	4	10-12	*
Bent over DB row	4	8-10	*
Seated cable row	4	8-10	*

Exercise	Sets	Reps	Rest
Standing BB curl	4	8-10	*
Seated DB curl	4	8-10	*

Wednesday & Saturday: Legs, Shoulders

Exercise	Sets	Reps	Rest
DB squats or goblet squats	4	8-10	*
Romanian deadlifts	4	8-10	*
DB lunges	4	8-10	*
Seated DB press	4	8-10	*
DB side raises	4	8-10	*
DB rear raises	4	8-10	*

HOME-BASED WORKOUT SCHEDULES

4-Day Workout Schedule (beginner)

Monday & Thursday: Chest, Back, Biceps and Triceps

Exercise	Sets	Reps	Rest
*DB bench press	4	8-10	*
Incline DB press	4	8-10	*
Bent-over BB row	3	8-10	*
Bent-over DB row	3	8-10	*
DB pullovers	3	10-12	*

Exercise			
Skull crushers (E-Z bar)	3	8-10	*
Bench dips	3	8-10	*
Standing BB curls	4	8-10	*

Tuesday & Friday: Legs, Shoulders and Abdominals

Exercise	Sets	Reps	Rest
DB squats or goblet squats	3	8-10	*
Romanian deadlifts	3	8-10	*
DB lunges	3	8-10	*
Seated DB press	4	8-10	*
DB side raises	4	8-10	*
Bicycle crossovers	3	15-20	*
V-ups	3	20-25	*

6-Day Workout Schedule (intermediate)

Monday & Thursday: Chest, Triceps, Abs

*Abdominal muscles worked 3x per week

Exercise	Sets	Reps	Rest
DB bench press	4	8-10	*
Incline DB press	4	8-10	*
DB fly	4	10-12	*
Skull crushers (E-Z bar)	4	8-10	*

Bench dips	4	10-12	*
Bicycle crossovers	3	15-20	*
V-ups	3	20-25	*
Reverse crunch w/stability ball	3	15-20	*

Tuesday & Friday: Back, Biceps

Exercise	Sets	Reps	Rest
DB pullovers	4	12-15	*
Bent over DB row	4	8-10	*
Bent over BB row	4	8-10	*
Standing BB curl	3	8-10	*
Seated DB curl	3	8-10	*

Wednesday & Saturday: Legs, Shoulders

Exercise	Sets	Reps	Rest
DB squats or goblets squats	4	8-10	*
Romanian deadlifts	4	8-10	*
DB lunges	4	8-10	*
Seated DB press	4	8-10	*
DB side raises	4	8-10	*
DB rear raises	4	8-10	*

ALTERNATIVE EXERCISES

There are often exercises an individual can't properly perform, perhaps due to injury or because that particular movement doesn't work well for him or her. If you encounter this issue, choose an alternative exercise to replace the one that's a problem.

Don't, however, make up an excuse to not perform an exercise simply because it's physically challenging for you and requires a lot of energy to perform, such as squats. Those exercises are both effective and necessary. Avoiding an exercise for unwarranted reasons only robs you of getting superior results in a search to find an easier way out.

Notice that I've included pull-ups in every back routine. I'm well aware that most people can't perform one pull-up, but the exercise is so beneficial that I recommend everyone include it in their routine and perform with a band for assistance if needed.

> If you do decide to choose an alternative exercise to replace one that's in your workout, make sure that it targets the same body part and is at the same level of difficulty as the one you're avoiding.

FULL-BODY WORKOUTS

Can you work out your entire body during one workout session? The short answer is yes, you can. However, there's a "but…"

Many programs that market their workouts based on three workouts per week use a full-body workout method of training. It's a quick and easy marketing tactic because it's appealing to think you can go to the gym for 30 minutes three times per week and develop a great body. What they fail to explain is that the degree in which the individual muscle groups are stimulated is minimal, and therefore minimal changes are produced in the muscles.

Full-body workouts require you to work each muscle group during one session, which means training seven muscle groups. Some muscle groups require a larger volume of training than others, such as legs. If you were to train each muscle group with enough volume to cause release of the fat-burning hormones, you would have to perform more than 40 sets to properly work each body part—that's too many.

The body can only sustain training at a high level of intensity for so many sets during one workout period. After about 25 sets, you begin to feel fatigued and your energy levels wane so you're not giving it your all. That's why it's not advisable to try to work out every body part during one workout session. I firmly believe there's a minimal stimulus that must be provided to the muscles of the body in order for muscular development to occur. This is precisely why a split workout is so effective with weight training routines.

By breaking up the body into two or three separate workouts, each workout can be performed with higher intensity and strength.

Nutrition & Meal Planning

Nutrition is the cornerstone for a lean and defined body. Your eating habits will completely make or break your success with fat loss and developing a defined body. Nutrition is so important that 75% of my system is comprised of it.

Nutritional strategies for lean body development have been my specialty for the past decade as I've devoted more and more time developing my system. I can't tell you how few people—even avid gym enthusiasts—don't understand how to apply certain principles of nutrition to achieve a lean and defined body. Nowhere does this lack of understanding occur more than in the supplement industry, where its existence depends on gimmicks and deception. The only exceptions to the gimmicks are food supplements such as protein powders and amino acids—which I consider to be food, not supplements. Nonetheless, I still advocate eating food over consuming food supplements.

Meal planning in my program revolves around three meals and two snacks per day. Research indicates that neither theory of eating six small meals a day or intermittent fasting is superior for fat loss. Thus, I've prepared a three meal, two snack schedule because I believe it's the best overall approach for the largest percent of the population. However, feel free to follow the eating schedule that works for you. If you feel that you'll do better eating six smaller meals per day, go for it. Everyone is different, and some people like the smaller, more frequent meals. For me, eating small, frequent meals doesn't provide the satiety of having a full meal, so I prefer the three meals and two snacks schedule. Regardless of the schedule you choose, what matters is your total daily caloric intake. Don't fret over eating in the evening, but *do* consider your daily allowance.

GETTING USED TO HEALTHY EATING

Some of you will want to start full-force into my healthy eating system while others might prefer to take things one or two steps at a time. As long as you continue to put the 9 principles into action, you'll be on the right track. In that respect, if you know you're someone that starts programs strong with good intentions, but later falls off the wagon because you were too aggressive, I recommend you start slower.

Eat a large green salad *every day*. The salad should have a minimum of three vegetables in it. For example, choose your base lettuce such as a dark green spinach or kale, and then add tomato, broccoli, and mushrooms. It doesn't matter which vegetables you choose, only that you include several in your salad. If you don't like salad, make sure you are at least getting those three large servings of vegetables.

HOW TO USE THE MASTER GROCERY LIST AND RECIPES

You've already been introduced to the MGL, and you're ready to shop. But first, you should know how to get the most out of it.

As you look at the sample 7-day fat loss nutrition plan in Appendix B, notice that—though the meals are broken down into the traditional groups of breakfast, lunch, and dinner—all meals are interchangeable. There's no set rule that you have to eat any of these foods at a specific time. In fact, you can eat breakfast for dinner and dinner for breakfast if you prefer. Any diet that has ridiculous rules about when you must consume certain foods is a complete gimmick.

After you've determined your list of meals, take note of the individual food items required to make these meals and mark these food items on the MGL so you can appropriately purchase these foods at the supermarket. Note: all vegetables are accepted—even if you don't see it listed on the MGL. Feel free to incorporate whatever you'd like.

VARIETY OF FOODS IN MEAL PLANNING

Having a small, simple list of foods for preparing your meals is something all lean athletes and fitness models have in common with their diets. Minimalism is a great tool to use in all areas of life, but is perhaps most helpful to practice when maintaining a lean and healthy body.

Part of the massive confusion that exists today with people wanting to know exactly what to eat is the vast variety of foods to choose from. In order to be successful in the long term, you must narrow your menu down to a couple handfuls of meals. If you haven't already done so, mark the foods on the MGL that you prefer so you'll be able to create at least a dozen different meals with these foods.

I mentioned earlier that you eat less variety in your diet than you are aware. We are truly creatures of habit. The average person eats the same thing every day for breakfast and only rotates a few different meals for lunches and dinners. Even when people eat out at restaurants, they often order the same meal every time. I highly recommend you decide on a core group of meals and stick with these.

> Never choose a food item or meal simply because it's healthy, if you don't actually like the food. You will *never* stick to a program if you don't enjoy the foods you eat to some degree.

If, for example, you absolutely hate salad, you can instead choose other vegetables that provide the same healthy, cancer-fighting phytochemicals such as broccoli, cauliflower, cabbage, or many other healthy vegetables. Since I've carefully chosen some of the most nutrient-dense foods on the planet, you can be assured you'll be getting all of the required nutrients the body needs for great health.

You will be amazed at how this method of meal planning positively affects you in several ways. Not only does it make it easy for you to plan your meals, but it also makes grocery shopping and calorie counting a cinch because you'll have the information memorized and stored in your brain in just a matter of weeks. Having too many choices for anything in life can result in confusion and indecisiveness. After conducting several surveys on why people don't eat healthy, I noticed that "not knowing how to cook" and "too much work" were at the top of the list. By following my system of preparing food in advance and creating your list of favorite meals, your chances for success are greatly increased. You now have a blueprint for taking action and putting this knowledge to work.

How to build healthy meals

Here are the guidelines we will use to construct healthy, fat-burning meals:

1) Pick a lean protein for each meal
2) Pick a green leafy salad for lunch or dinner
3) Pick a vegetable for every meal
4) Pick a complex starchy carb for lunch and dinner
5) Pick a fruit for breakfast
6) Pick a healthy fat for every meal

7) Pick two between-meal snacks

We begin each meal by choosing a lean protein such as chicken breast. Constructing your meals always revolves around the choice of protein. Second, we choose a vegetable or salad such as a cabbage and broccoli salad. In this case we would add the fat with crushed walnuts and honey yogurt dressing in the cabbage salad. Then we would add a baked yam for the starchy complex carb to complete the meal. Remember, salads can be freely eaten without concern for quantity. Multiple vegetables can also be eaten in your salad or raw or steamed as a side dish.

For breakfast, three egg whites and one yolk scrambled with mushrooms and tomatoes could be your lean protein with vegetables, and a cup of steel cut oatmeal with a handful of blueberries sweetened with natural Stevia as your complex carb and fruit.

Snacks are usually saved for mid-afternoon and after dinner, depending on the individual. One example of a good snack is non-fat Greek yogurt with some vanilla protein powder mixed in and a tablespoon of walnuts or pecans sprinkled on top. Another one might be a berry protein shake with blueberries, strawberries, protein powder, and almond milk with Stevia natural sweetener.

By following this meal-builder template and paying attention to portions of proteins and condiments used for salads, you'll automatically be near the total amount of calories and macronutrients that you should reach each day for goals of fat loss.

One nice thing about the MGL is that you can take any of these foods and plug them into your meals according to the guidelines above. The quantities of food are determined from your calculations of weight, activity level, and goals for your fat loss. A smaller female will be consuming lean protein portions around 4 ounces per serving, whereas a larger male will consume 8-ounce servings of lean protein. The food choices are the same for everyone, but the portions vary according to the individual.

A question I'm often asked about how I've laid out meal building is whether or not you absolutely have to choose a food from each of the categories listed. No, you do not—but there are a few rules that should be adhered to as often as possible:

1) Always choose a lean protein for every meal as the cornerstone for everything else. It's not a good practice to consume carbs

alone unless they are of the complex, fibrous nature such as salads and vegetables. Maintaining stable blood glucose levels and minimizing the insulin response are important factors for reducing fat storage.

2) Consuming green salads and vegetables on a daily basis is crucial for overall health, and is very helpful to your efforts for developing a lean body. If there were only two groups of food I could consume for the rest of my life it would be lean proteins and green salads with other varieties of vegetables.

3) Snacks can be very helpful in preventing cravings that result in making poor food choices. By having healthy snacks readily available during times of temptation, you'll prevent the potential derailment of your program.

Most people have little knowledge of how to navigate around the kitchen—this is especially true for some men. As part of your learning process, start with basic meals where you simply cook foods separately; later, you can work your way toward more complicated recipes. I personally strive to keep my recipes very simple and rarely make meals that require more than five different ingredients. I don't have the patience to deal with long lists of instructions, and I'm guessing that many of you would agree.

Here is the sequence of tasks I've used to make progress in the kitchen:

1) Get familiar with all the foods on the MGL
2) Make your list of favorite foods to use for the meals you'll create
3) Learn how to use your favorite foods to create meals that are appealing
4) Begin experimenting with more advanced recipes using the same foods

ADVANCED FOOD PREPARATION

Implementing the advanced food preparation system

In Principle 6, we discussed the importance of having food prepared in advance in order to save time and have food readily available. I can't stress enough how important this will be to your success. Take the time to prepare food during two sessions of the week and you'll save hours of time cooking your meals.

Every meal in my recipe guide can be prepared in 10 minutes or less. When I developed my recipe list and constructed my meals, quick preparation was the second-most important factor (next to choosing fresh, healthy ingredients) for getting lean. Survey after survey indicates that a shortage of time is the number one reason why people don't cook meals at home. Solving this problem is the most important factor if you want to be lean and healthy. There's no way around it.

Preparation of vegetables and produce

You should already know which food items you need for your meals, so now you can start cleaning, cutting, and bagging your vegetables for easy retrieval for your salads. For example, if you're including broccoli, cauliflower, and cabbage, take these items and cut them into smaller pieces and place into baggies or in Tupperware containers.

Make sure the vegetables are laid out on a towel after washing so they can dry a bit before placing into storage. If you eat one large salad per day you'll only need enough for three to four salads. This isn't very much, so you'll have to get used to the quantity you prepare each session.

For those of you who don't like raw vegetables, still perform the same cleaning, cutting and bagging process, but when it comes time to prepare your salad, place the vegetables to be steamed into a Zip n' Steam bag for a couple of minutes. Word to the wise: with the exception of Brussels sprouts, steaming vegetables before storing them in the refrigerator is not good. The vegetables won't stay fresh, and you don't want that.

Vegetables such as tomatoes are not supposed to be cut and refrigerated, so they must be left until you're ready to prepare your salad.

Today, consumers have many choices in the supermarket. If you refuse to wash and cut your vegetables, the next best option is to purchase pre-washed and cut vegetables. They are more expensive and not quite as healthy, but if this is a deal-breaker for you then take this route. Believe me, I can relate to the fact that no one wants to spend more time than necessary preparing food. We all have busy schedules, and adding additional work to an already busy schedule is not in the cards for most people. By using this system, you'll save hours of time per week. If you think its quicker picking up take-out food or eating out at restaurants, think again. Once you consider the time it takes traveling to the restaurant and waiting for your food, you'll see that you don't actually save time.

Know this: no matter how fast you can get take-out food, you don't stand a chance of getting lean by eating it. Regardless of where you eat, you're in a place where you have no control over the method of food preparation. Restaurant food is loaded with calories and sodium—at least twice that of a home-cooked meal that uses the same ingredients.

Preparation of protein-rich foods: meats, fish, and eggs

The most time-consuming part of cooking involves cooking your protein sources. I've developed some very efficient strategies for preparing proteins without sacrificing the quality of the meal.

Some foods lend themselves well for cooking in advance— others don't. It also depends on how fussy of a person you are. I know people who won't eat a meal unless it's cooked at that moment, whereas other people don't care if it was leftovers from five days ago. Personally, I'm kind of between the two extremes. As long as the food isn't altered in taste or consistency, I'm fine with cooking in advance. The good thing is, the majority of the protein sources cooked in advance from the MGL turn out well. The only protein I prefer to cook at the moment I eat is fish. Since fish is only cooked for about 10 minutes, the preparation time for meals stays within our limit of 10 minutes or less.

There are exceptions to even that, however. There's nothing wrong with cooking salmon in advance, for example, because it goes very well on top of a kale salad with crushed pecans. It also depends on how you will serve your fish. If it's used in your salad, then cooking in advance works well; if you plan on eating it as your main dish with steamed asparagus, I recommend cooking it at the moment you prepare your meal.

Methods of cooking proteins

My favorite method of cooking any meat is with a crock pot, also called a slow cooker. The meat turns out very tender, and you can cook up to several pounds of meat at a time with no mess to clean-up afterwards. I highly recommend purchasing a simple, inexpensive crock pot for less than $40. By using a crock pot, you could even turn it on

94

before going to bed, or when you leave for work in the morning. Eight hours later, it's done. All you add is water to cover the top of the meat and any herbs and spices you like.

The other often-used method of cooking meats is in a skillet, which is how I cook chicken breasts. I prefer chicken breast cooked this way when I eat Italian-style dishes, which I do at least twice per week. Cooking meats in two different ways provides for more variety with meals and tastes better, depending on what you're combining it with.

Eggs are the other essential protein that is nice to have prepared in advance. There are countless ways to serve eggs, but the two easiest ways to have pre-cooked eggs on hand are to hard-boil them or cook them in a muffin pan. Take a muffin pan and give a quick spray to the pan with coconut oil. Then crack open an egg and place it in each muffin place for the desired number of eggs you want cooked for storage. Place the pan in the oven at 350 degrees for 25 minutes until the egg is fully cooked. Allow to cool and remove to store in a Tupper ware container. These can be used in so many ways; you could eat them for breakfast or crumble them up and add them to a salad for lunch or dinner.

DESSERTS & SNACKS

The list of snacks and desserts I've created in my recipe guide all consist of protein and carbs. Most other desserts are of the simple sugar-based types, which are not good for keeping insulin levels in check. By adding protein to the desserts on my list via a half-scoop of protein powder and using Greek yogurt versus regular yogurt, the release of insulin into the blood is somewhat reduced. You will have yourself a healthy, low-sugar, high-protein dessert or snack when the urge hits you. This helps prevent glucose from being stored in fat cells as excess calories. You could even use any one of the dessert or snack options for a quick on-the-go breakfast in place of the breakfast choices listed, too.

Going to bed on an empty stomach is something very difficult for me to do. It's a nightly ritual for me to make one of these desserts before going to bed, and it helps me to sleep better as a result. Eating before bedtime does not lead to weight gain; that is a common myth. Research has indicated conclusively that it makes no difference what time of day calories are consumed.

PROTEIN PORTIONS AND WEIGHING FOODS

After you've cooked your proteins, the meats should be weighed out in 4, 6, or 8-ounce portions and placed in sandwich bags for quick retrieval. That way you know exactly how much protein you're consuming and your total number of calories. The size in which you should measure your protein portions out to depends on your body weight. You will know after a short while what is appropriate for you.

The number one reason we have such rampant problems with obesity in the U.S. is because people consume way more than they should. I mentioned earlier that studies indicate people consume 40% more than they think they're eating, on average. As you begin this healthy eating program, I want you to know what proper quantities of food you're consuming look like.

The only foods we don't have to be concerned with measuring are greens and individual vegetables. The calories from these foods contribute minimally to your overall totals. Even though you can eat as much of these foods as you want, it's still wise for you to have an understanding of portion size for the simple reason of knowing in case someone asks you the question.

FOOD TRACKING

The easiest way to keep track of your daily totals is to set up a free account on MyFitnessPal or another similar mobile app or website. Once you've added all the individual foods you eat, it becomes very easy to track all your macronutrients. This presents a system that's highly accurate for monitoring everything you eat, so there's no guesswork left for you to do.

In addition to downloading an app like MyFitnessPal or finding a good tracking system on a different website, purchase a cheap digital scale and some measuring cups. *Know your macronutrients.* You don't want to be guessing those figures. It only takes about 30 minutes to add up all your foods and you're done. Simply enter what you ate for a meal and the app indicates exactly where you're at for the day with all your numbers. You will learn a lot by doing this, and, after you have a good grasp on understanding macronutrients in foods, you won't have to continue recording totals.

DETERMINING TOTAL DAILY CALORIC INTAKE

The total number of calories you consume on a daily basis is the most important number you'll need in determining how to reduce body fat. Anyone telling you that calories don't matter doesn't understand *The Law of Energy Balance,* which (in its simplest form) looks like this:

Energy in = Energy out + Change in Body Stores

This is simply another way to state the law of basic thermodynamics, since energy can't be created or destroyed. All energy *must* be accounted for in some form. In this case, differences between intake and output show up as changes in the energy stores of the body.

Changes in energy stores will show up as changes in the amount of different tissues in the body as indicated on the right side of this equation. Excess energy from calories is converted or stored into additional body tissue such as body fat or lean muscle mass, depending on the activities of the person. If you're engaging in a serious daily workout routine such as one of the routines I've recommended, more of the excess calories consumed will be used to build lean muscle tissue, whereas someone that's sedentary will likely see increases in body fat due to reduced energy expenditure.

> In order to lose weight, you must burn more calories than you consume over a given period of time. Conversely, you must consume more calories than you burn over a given period of time to gain weight.

It doesn't matter if the source of calories is healthy or unhealthy; a surplus is a surplus, and you will increase body fat even if you eat healthy. This is a fact that too many people don't consider when following a fat loss program. Consuming the correct number of calories to achieve your goal requires some feedback on your part so you can make adjustments according to your results. By doing so, you will find the optimal number based on your body's requirements.

In order to make this as easy as possible, I've included a simple method of determining calorie intake for fat loss below. Remember, it's critical to understand calories and the macronutrients that contribute to those calories—there's no better time to learn about this topic than now.

Here are some ballpark figures for calorie requirements for men and women:

Men:
Fat loss: 2000-2500
Maintenance: 2600-2900

Women:
Fat loss: 1400-1800
Maintenance: 1900-2100

A more accurate way to calculate your daily caloric intake is the following:

Fat loss: 10-12 calories per lb. of body weight
Maintenance: 14-16 calories per lb. of body weight

Use the number 10 for a sedentary person, 11 for someone who participates in moderate activity, or 12 for a very active person.

Example: for a 190 lb. sedentary male: 10 x 190 lbs. = 1900 calories per day.

I've found this method to be quite accurate for the majority of people. You can at least start with these figures and see how you progress each week. If you're using the 12 multiplier and you're not losing fat, you need to reduce to 11 times your weight. Once you know approximately what your daily caloric intake should be, it's time to calculate the macronutrient ratios to determine grams of protein, carbs, and fat. Before you calculate your ratio, however, spend some time understanding macronutrients in general.

UNDERSTANDING THE MACRONUTRIENTS: PROTEIN, CARBS, AND FATS

Protein

Protein has always been the macronutrient most people concern themselves with. The building blocks of protein are 20 **amino acids** that are consumed from both animal and plant sources. Of the 20 amino acids, 9 are considered to be essential because they cannot be synthesized by the human body. The remaining other 11 amino acids are considered nonessential because the body has the necessary enzymes to synthesize these amino acids. From these 20 amino acids, all proteins of the body are manufactured. The difference in the function of each protein is determined by the sequence in which the chain of amino acids is arranged. This allows for an endless number of sequences to build different proteins in the body—for which there is an endless number of functions.

The reason we emphasize the consumption of protein at each meal is because—unlike carbs and fats—proteins can't be stored to any degree. There's only a small amount of amino acids circulating in the bloodstream and stored in various tissues of the body. Even so, it would take several days of not eating any protein before the body would deplete itself of stores.

The number one question asked related to macronutrients is: how much protein should I be eating to lose weight? The problem with this question is the way it's asked. The question is asked as though protein helps to lose weight, when in fact the only thing that results in weight loss is a calorie deficit (burning more calories than you currently consume). Protein does contribute more than carbs or fats to what's termed the **thermic effect of food** (TEF), but the difference is small when compared to overall calories consumed.

The TEF is the amount of energy that's expended in addition to a person's resting metabolic rate for the processing of food for use and storage. It's the energy used in digestion, absorption, and distribution of nutrients. It is one of the components of metabolism along with resting metabolic rate and the exercise component which determines your overall total energy requirements.

Protein shakes versus protein in foods

A common question: Is protein from a supplement superior to protein from foods?

The quick answer: no.

There is nothing magical about drinking a protein shake for enhancing muscle-building gains or fat loss. Any protein consumed over and above your body's requirements will end up as fat stored in the body just like extra carbs or fats would also be stored. Extra calories are extra calories, regardless of the macronutrient that contributed.

Your first choice of protein sources should *always* be through whole, natural foods. No food supplement will ever take the place that natural sources of amino acids found in whole foods take. Our body was meant to consume foods and will digest and utilize the amino acids of the proteins to the greatest extent through foods.

The sources of foods with the highest quality and bioavailability are from animals, eggs, fish, and dairy products. These are considered **complete proteins**—proteins that contain all the essential 20 amino acids your body requires.

Vegetarians can also consume the 20 amino acids required by the body from meatless sources, but this requires education beyond the scope of this book.

Carbs

We already mentioned in Principle 6 that carbs in general have been vilified, and the reason for this is because "good carbs" have been grouped together with "bad carbs," or processed carbs. Carbs are our body's preferred source of energy, and the brain functions solely on glucose which it gets from metabolizing carbs; so it's important not to exclude all types of carbs.

Let's try to make sense of the confusion so you can start making educated choices when building healthy meals. Just as there are different categories of fat, there are also different categories of carbs. The key is to learn which food sources provide the healthy carbs your body requires for optimal performance and daily functioning.

Carbs are usually broken down into two main categories based on how quickly they are metabolized. Generally speaking, there are simple carbs and complex carbs. These can be further classified, which we will do now.

Classification of Carbs

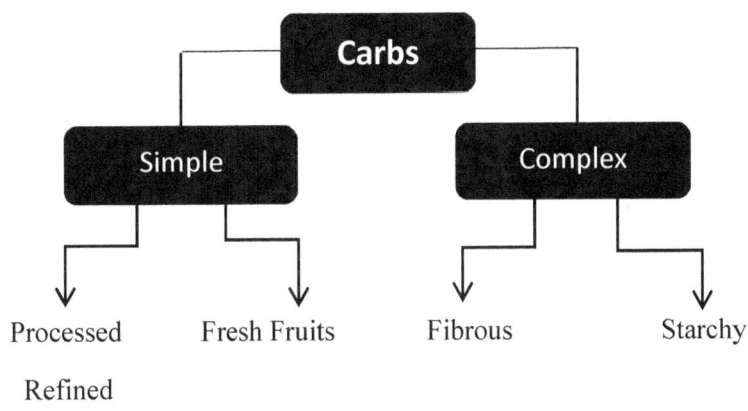

Simple carbs: Fast digesting, processed, or refined

These are bad carbs. They are often nutritionally void of nutrients and are loaded with empty calories. For ease of discussion, I will use the term *processed carbs.*

If someone were to ask me which foods I believe contribute to our nation's obesity epidemic the most, I would undoubtedly say "foods made with processed carbs." It's more than a coincidence that processed carbs are where the big money is in the food manufacturing industry. Boxed and packaged foods, for the most part, are completely processed carbs. That is why you should consider almost everything found in a box or package a poor source of nutrients and loaded with carbs that will greatly contribute to gaining fat.

Food manufacturers often fool people into thinking that an unhealthy food is healthy because they add a certain nutrient to make it appear nutritious. The term "fortified" is frequently used to indicate a certain nutrient has been added to the product. We should not view foods as mere vitamins or minerals in an isolated way. This is not what nutrition is about. Food in its natural state is very complex and can't be reproduced in a lab or food manufacturing facility. The enormous array of other nutrients and phytochemicals, which we don't even completely understand, resides in natural food. The synergistic interplay of thousands of molecules through complex biochemical processes is what provides the *real* benefits of eating a diet filled with fresh, natural fruits and vegetables.

Don't fall for the gimmicky products that add a nutrient such as omega-3 to a packaged food in an attempt to make it appear healthy. It's wiser to choose foods that are naturally healthy and are considered nutrient dense such as those found on my MGL.

Processed carbs to avoid

- Most breads
- White rice
- Cakes
- Pies
- Muffins
- Boxed cereals
- Cookies
- Candy, milk chocolate
- Crackers & chips, pretzels
- All Desserts
- Pancakes & waffles
- Breaded Foods
- Pastas, Noodles
- Jelly
- Bagels
- Pizza
- Energy Bars, Granola Bars
- Ketchup
- Sweetened yogurts
- Soda
- Canned items with sugar listed in the top 3 ingredients
- Honey, agave
- Corn syrup
- Brown sugar
- Molasses

- Fructose (except naturally occurring in fresh fruits)
- Maltose
- Dextrose
- Fruit Juice concentrates (Natural fruit juice is occasionally acceptable in small quantities for cooking)

Let's look at the one exception of a simple carb that *should* be included in your diet: fresh fruits. This is a topic that causes a lot of confusion.

Fruits are in the category of simple carbs because they are quickly digested; this is so their component sugars (fructose) are readily available for energy needs of the body. Fruits—unlike other simple sugars—are nutrient-dense foods that support good health. They also differ from other simple carbs in their high fiber content. The fibrous bulk of the fruit provides bulk to the stool for digestive tract health.

Additionally, many fruits contain **phytonutrients** that are known for their cancer-fighting properties that can only be matched by certain vegetables. Water content is another differentiating factor of fruit. Any sugars found in fruit are highly diluted, which minimizes the spike that usually occurs with other simple sugars found in processed carbs. Besides that, I've never seen anyone get fat from eating fresh fruits.

Complex carbs: Slow digesting

These are good carbs. Complex carbs can be further divided into **fibrous carbs** and **starchy carbs**.

Fibrous carbs are, as the name suggests, high in fiber content. This is because plants are mostly indigestible and pass through the digestive tract without the body extracting much in the way of calories. Due to the transit time of these foods passing along the intestinal tract, plant foods are known for reducing the chance of developing gastrointestinal diseases such as colon cancer. The fiber consumption of the average American is low, and many researchers believe low fiber intake is a significant reason for the high cancer rate among Americans.

If you had to choose one category of food to accompany lean protein for good health, I'd recommend eating a diet high in plant foods consisting of green, leafy salad and cruciferous vegetables. Numerous studies have analyzed the diets of groups of individuals in the regions of the world with the longest average life spans. They've found that the consumption of high quantities of vegetables was a common factor found in all groups. These regions around the world are referred to as the "Blue Zones." Here are the five zones that are included on Dan Buettner's list in his book, *The Blue Zones*:

Okinawa, Japan
Sardinia, Italy
Loma Linda, California
Nicoya, Costa Rica
Ikaria, Greece

If I could instruct you to do one thing in your diet, it would be to eliminate processed or refined carbs and replace them with complex fibrous carbs from plant foods. Not only have fibrous carbs been found to decrease several major forms of cancer and reduce diabetes through increasing insulin sensitivity, but they greatly help you with fat loss.

The low calorie content—yet bulky nature—of the plants help offer a feeling of satiety and may cause a decrease in appetite-stimulating hormones. For the most part, it's nearly impossible to eat too many calories from plant foods—which make this group of food an indispensable part of your diet.

List of complex fibrous carbs

- Asparagus
- Brussels sprouts
- Broccoli
- Bell peppers
- Bok Choy
- Cucumber
- Cauliflower
- Carrots
- Celery
- Cabbage (red + green)
- Green beans
- Kohlrabi
- Lettuce (all types)
- Mushrooms
- Rutabaga

- Turnips
- Tomatoes
- Kale
- Onions
- Spinach
- Peas
- Zucchini

Starchy complex carbs are the other sub-category of complex carbs. **Starches** are long, complex chains called polysaccharides made up of simple carbs. They are completely digestible and therefore absorbed by the body, whereas the fibrous carbs are not absorbed. The assimilation and absorption process with starchy carbs occurs at a much slower rate than with simple carbs, therefore providing you with a more sustained source of energy and a feeling of satiety for a longer period of time.

Although many of the starchy carbs are loaded with nutrients, they are much denser in calories than fibrous carbs; they should therefore be limited for anyone following a fat-loss program. The foods that I've found to be the best starchy carbs to incorporate into a diet are yams and sweet potatoes, beans, lentils and steel-cut oatmeal. The remaining foods don't provide enough nutrients for the amount of calories they contain.

Common complex starchy carbs

- Yam
- Sweet potato
- Squash
- Oatmeal
- Quinoa
- Brown rice
- Lentils
- Beans
- Corn
- Whole grain breads
- Whole grain pastas
- Whole grain cereals

A word about the Glycemic Index

I can't tell you the number of times I've been asked about a food's ranking on the glycemic index. The **glycemic index** was created for those with blood sugar issues, such as diabetics, and should *not* be used to make decisions on whether a food should be included in a diet.

For example, carrots rank relatively high on the index, yet are low in calories. Carrots are very nutritious and provide a lot of fiber; they should *not* be excluded from the diet because of their ranking.

Use common sense. We should be concentrating on the *important* questions about what we consume, such as whether the food we're about to eat naturally occurs in plants, or if it is a processed, calorie-dense food.

Fats

Fats were once perceived as negatively as carbs are today. For more than two decades we were told by health officials and the media that heart disease was caused by high-fat diets.

Similar theories have attempted to make eggs look like a food to avoid. For almost 40 years eggs were considered an unhealthy food based on the following assumptions:

- Eggs contain saturated fats
- Dietary saturated fat from food becomes cholesterol (lipids) in the body and leads to high blood cholesterol
- Increased levels of cholesterol lead to higher rates of heart attacks and strokes
- Consuming fat makes you fat

Scientist Ancel Keys was a significant contributor to this false theory. He believed there was a relationship between fat consumption and high blood cholesterol. From this, he developed what was known as "The Seven Country Study," which demonstrated the correlation between dietary fat consumption and heart disease. His theory was later known as the lipid hypothesis (which we discussed in Principle 5) and became widely accepted in the medical establishment around 1965. Health officials in the government jumped on this bandwagon, developing policies and guidelines that steered people away from fats and the consumption of meats. After that, the government instructed

106

people to minimize their consumption of eggs.

As a result of the reduction in calories from protein sources like fatty meats, consumers were encouraged to eat more grains and cereals to increase their carb intake. In the '80s, the food pyramid was revised and people were instructed to consume up to 12 servings of grains a day. The only large study using a low-fat diet to show a reduction in heart disease involved the use of statins (drugs like Lipitor), so advocating the lipid hypothesis became attractive to drug companies producing statins. As of today, these drugs have been the biggest blockbuster selling drugs ever in the history of the pharmaceutical industry; they garner profits in the *tens of billions*.

Even though Americans reduced their fat intake, the rate of obesity and diabetes has exploded, and many health professionals attribute this to the increase in consumption of carbohydrates. The problem with Keys's research was that he only used data from the countries that supported his theory while failing to include the two countries that didn't. The study was a fraud, yet the government and media quickly ran with the study's results and created the following guidelines (introduced to the public by the United States Department of Agriculture around 1977):

1) Reduce consumption of fat and cholesterol
2) Increase consumption of complex carbs like grains, fruits and vegetables
3) Reduce consumption of refined and processed sugars

And so was born a low-fat, high-carb diet for all of Americans to follow. Notice, reading the chart below, that this was about the time the rise of obesity and increase of Type 2 diabetes in America began.

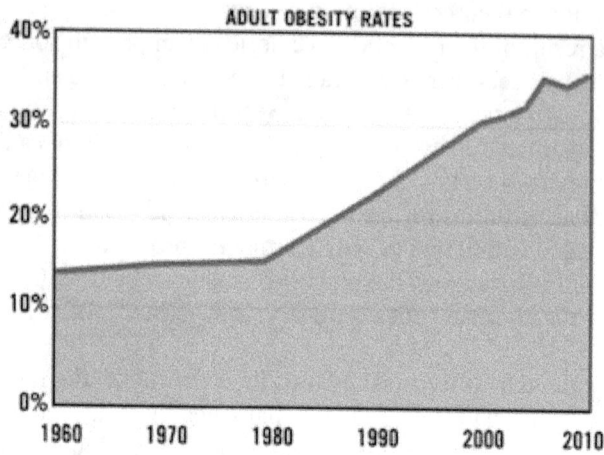

Much of the data refuting the Keys research has been out there for a long time, but it took a lot of effort to break down resistance. Too many parties benefited—particularly financially—from the consensus of Keys's study. Doctors and scientists that backed Keys's research were hesitant to change their minds in spite of the new findings. After more improvements in technology developed, there were finally enough experts that stood up and said "no, the consensus is wrong."

Today, there's a new understanding of the role of fats and cholesterol in the diet. Generally speaking, certain types of fats ("good fats") are now better known as playing a healthy role. Also, the understanding of how the body transforms dietary fat to cholesterol has been radically changed. The previous models, which put the blame on saturated fats contributing to higher levels of dangerous **low-density lipoproteins** (LDL), have been thrown out.

The truth about eggs and cholesterol

- Most cholesterol in our blood is produced by our liver. Diet has a very small effect on the overall level of cholesterol with an exception of roughly 5% of the population.
- Cholesterol is essential for many biological processes of the body including: cell membranes, hormone production, and bile for the liver to digest fats. Cholesterol is measured by the amount of lipoproteins in the blood. Lipoproteins are the carriers of cholesterol.

- LDL, sometimes inaccurately labeled as "bad cholesterol," carry cholesterol through the blood to cells to perform its jobs.
- Animal fats, like those contained in eggs, are composed of cholesterol and triglycerides. These are the main lipids we consume. **Triglycerides** are compounds consisting of three molecules of fatty acids esterified to glycerol and stored in adipose (fat) cells.
- High levels of LDL or triglycerides can be an indicator that the body is producing or has too much cholesterol.
- High levels of cholesterol in the blood may contribute to the formation of plaques in the blood vessels and cause heart disease.
- **High-density lipoproteins** (HDL) carry cholesterol away from blood vessels back to the liver for processing. That is why it is called good cholesterol (even though it's incorrect to label as such).
- Even though egg yolks are high in fat, only 27% of the fat is saturated; the rest is **polyunsaturated fat**, which contains HDL and has been shown to improve the ratio between HDL and LDL.
- Several large studies have recently shown no correlation between consuming half a dozen eggs per week and heart disease.

Classification of fats: Saturated & Unsaturated

Saturated fats are mainly derived from animal fats such as beef, pork, poultry, and milk. Examples of other saturated fats are coconut oil and palm oil. These are examples of fats we've been taught to reduce in the diet, but for the wrong reason (as previously discussed). Reducing consumption of saturated fats in your diet doesn't translate into lower blood cholesterol levels. The reason for reducing saturated fats is because they don't provide the essential fatty acids the body requires for important biological processes.

Unsaturated fats are derived from plants and vegetables. These fats are further categorized into *mono-* and *polyunsaturated fats*, depending on their molecular structure and chemical properties. Some examples of both mono- and polyunsaturated fats are: olive oil, walnuts, avocado, and fish oil. These fats are considered healthy fats because they possess certain healthy properties that protect the heart. Because of these properties, they are classified as **essential fatty acids**, or, EFAs. Our bodies simply cannot produce EFAs. Just like the requirement of essential amino acids from the diet we discussed in proteins, EFAs must also come from our diet. Not only must they be supplied by our diet, but they also need to be in the correct ratios.

Essential Fatty Acids: Omega-3 & Omega-6

These two EFAs are also referred to as **alpha-linolenic acid** (LNA) and **linoleic acid** (LA), respectively. These are fats we need to concern ourselves with when creating a healthy, sustainable, fat-burning diet. Saturated fats are difficult to completely avoid, but should be reduced to a minimum because they are nutritionally void other than providing protein. The unsaturated fats that contain the proper ratios of EFAs should be the focus when examining fats in the diet.

I'll never forget a statistic that stuck with me from when I was in elementary school while watching a film in class called *Nanook of the North*. I learned (and later looked at some research to support it) that Eskimos consumed a high-fat diet almost exclusively of whale blubber and fish. So essentially, they consumed fats primarily comprised of omega-3 fatty acids. The astonishing fact is that the Eskimos' rates of heart disease and strokes are extremely low compared to the rates amongst average Americans—which supports the findings that not all fats are bad. Not only do some fats *not* contribute to heart disease, but they have powerful cardio-protective properties that prevent heart disease.

A noteworthy distinction to make with these two EFAs is that the ratio in the diet has gotten completely out of whack over the past couple decades. A healthy ratio of the EFAs is believed to be around 2:1 (omega-6: omega-3), which is close in line of that which we evolved. Today, in the Western world, the ratio is more like 20:1. The primary reason for this disproportionate ratio is due to the high consumption of grains and grain-fed animal meats we consume. This is why I'm an advocate for consuming grass-fed beef whenever possible; the omega-6 fats end up in the tissues of the animal because they are fed grain instead of grass and plants. Grass contains much higher quantities of omega-3 fats.

Some benefits of omega-3s:

- Improved blood cholesterol

110

- Helps prevent diabetes
- Regulates important physiological functions like blood pressure, blood clotting
- Reduces depression
- Increases bone strength
- Protects against dementia and Alzheimer's
- Slows the aging process

A list of unsaturated EPAs:

- Olive oil
- Almonds & almond butter
- Macadamia nuts
- Avocado
- Pecans
- Walnuts
- Flaxseed
- Fish oil
- Pine nuts
- Hemp seeds

Fish oils

Eating fatty fish is the best way to get your supply of two specific omega-3 fats: **Eicosapentaenoic acid** (EPA) and **docosahexaenoic acid** (DHA). These fats are found in salmon, sardines, herring, tuna, trout, and mackerel.

There are certain nuts that are also good sources of omega-3 fats such as flax seed and walnuts.

Hydrogenated fats & Trans-fatty acids

These are the fats to avoid at all costs. By avoiding processed, packaged foods, your chances of eliminating these fats from the diet will be greatly increased. Hydrogenated (and partially hydrogenated) fats are commonly found in baked products to increase shelf life and prevent spoiling. The problem is, the preservation of the product has the reverse effect on our health.

Here is a list of foods to avoid which contain trans-fatty acids:

- Chips*
- Crackers*
- Cakes, pies, pastries & doughnuts
- Refined vegetable oils
- Margarine
- Shortening
- Fried foods (all fast food items, French fries, meats)

*Not all of these foods are produced with trans-fatty acids in them anymore. Most food manufacturers have taken steps to eliminate or greatly reduce the amount of these fats in their products.

The effects from eating products containing these fats are serious and shouldn't be taken lightly. We can get by some "no-no's" in our diets without suffering too many bad consequences, but consuming trans-fatty acids and hydrogenated fats is *not* one of them.

***

We've talked a lot about fats. Here's a summary of the important guidelines to follow while you create your meals and follow the macronutrient ratios with protein, carbs, and fats:

1) Look to unsaturated fats that contain the EFAs when calculating your fat intake
2) Consume approximately 20-30% of your total calories in unsaturated fats
3) Minimize the amount of animal fat by choosing lean cuts of meats
4) Avoid fried foods like the plague
5) Stick with low-fat dairy products like milk, cheese, and yogurt
6) Consume fatty sources of fish with high levels of DHA and EPA oils
7) Purchase grass-fed beef whenever possible
8) Keep in mind that although nuts are healthy fats, they're high in calories
9) Use olive oil and coconut oil sprays for cooking to reduce calorie consumption

DETERMINING YOUR MACRONUTRIENT RATIOS

If you don't remember the lesson in Principle 6, now is a good time to go back and review the material and look at the macronutrient graphic.

In order to calculate your macronutrient ratios, you'll need the following conversions:

1 gram of protein = 4 calories
1 gram of carbs = 4 calories
1 gram of fat = 9 calories

There is no such thing as an optimal macronutrient ratio to follow that can be applied to everyone. These ratios vary within a wide range depending on a person's level of body fat, activity level, and sensitivity to glucose. The recommendations I make should be adjusted according to your personal profile and goals for losing body fat.

Here are some guidelines to help you choose macronutrient ratios to follow when creating your meal plan:

- Maximum fat loss: 45-50% protein, 25-30% carbs, 25% fats

This is ideal for those with body fat levels over 35% who are inactive and sensitive to carbs. Fat stores typically are located on the belly in males, and the belly, hips, and thighs in females. Reducing carbs to less than 25% is too uncomfortable, so I don't recommend it. Very low carb diets are not sustainable, and I don't advocate them.

- Moderate fat loss: 40% protein, 30% carbs, 30% fats

This is ideal for individuals who are inactive, but not obese. I find this ratio to be very effective for the widest range of individuals for losing body fat. This is also the ratio I follow when reducing body fat to extremely low levels. It's easy to follow and doesn't feel overly depriving.

- Maintenance of body fat levels: 30% protein, 50% carbs, 20% fats

This is ideal for those who have lost body fat and want to maintain current levels. If you think you are sensitive to carbs and tend to increase fat quickly, reduce your carbs by 5-10%. That will also require you to increase your protein and fat slightly to maintain total calories.

DETERMINING THE PROPER RATE OF FAT LOSS

The best way to lose body fat and keep it off for good is to do it at a rate that doesn't cause you to sacrifice lean muscle tissue or trigger a physiological state of starvation. Most people that fail are much too aggressive in the beginning and want immediate, quick results. What good is it if your weight loss ends up being temporary?

A realistic amount of fat to lose is 1% of your body weight per week.

Oftentimes you'll hear people quoting two pounds per week is the target weight to lose, but this can be a drastically different percentage on a person that's 325 pounds versus someone that's 125 pounds. A larger person is going to lose significantly more weight than a smaller person, so using percentages is a better approach.

For a 300-pound person, 1% translates to a loss of 3 pounds per week. In reality, you will experience a larger than 1% drop in weight in the beginning, even without using drastic measures. This is a result of eliminating so many excess processed carbs that tend to hold large volumes of water in the body. Don't get the false impression in the first couple of weeks that all your weight loss is fat, because it's not.

Fat loss is not linear. It's not an exact science that follows precise laws like mathematics, but there *are* definite rules that apply to everyone. You may experience weeks where the scale does not change and other times when you drop a couple weeks' worth of weight. Don't get too hung up with the numbers in the beginning; your body is making some adjustments and will provide you with more accurate feedback within a couple weeks. Your main objective is to follow your eating plan and continue your workout schedule.

Don't look at your fat loss as a project that has a beginning or an end. Instead, learn the principles and practices of the leanest, most successful people in the world and make this a lifestyle that you live by on a daily basis. That way, if you have a bad day or week where you skip workouts or eat poorly, you're less likely to beat yourself up and quit. You won't "quit" anything that you'll be doing for the rest of your life. If you fall off the track, you simply get back to living your new lifestyle habits. By looking at these nutritional changes as your new *lifestyle*, your mind interprets the behavior more effectively than it would if you viewed them as a temporary diet.

Conclusion

I hope this book has helped you learn important principles to guide you in your quest for creating a healthy, lean, and muscular body.

This is a *lifestyle*. The word "lifestyle" implies something permanent. You don't have to think about what the next step in a plan is; the acts of exercise and nutrition each day should be effortless. There's no deadline; no sense of hurry or stress to get somewhere. If you falter in your healthy habits for a day here or there, simply pick yourself back up and follow the program you've established for your lifestyle.

When you've achieved your initial goals and lost the fat you've set out to lose, you can adjust your calories and macronutrients to a maintenance level and enjoy the best years of your life with great health.

Here's my guarantee to you: if you follow the 9 *HoffmanFit* principles diligently and are willing to put forth the work and dedication towards your goal, you'll witness incredible changes to your body that you've never seen before. That means sticking with these principles for *at least* three months.

Procrastination is the killer of success. It robs you of so many valuable things in life. There are an endless number of excuses to delay achieving your goal, but I want you to remember a phrase that I often think of when making an excuse:

> "If it's important enough, you'll find a way to achieve the goal."

If you're ready to dramatically improve your health and fitness and want to receive more in-depth information, please visit http://www.hoffmanfit.com/ and subscribe to my FREE blog updates and newsletter. Several times per month you'll receive fat loss tips, workout strategies, and quick and tasty recipes ideas to help you reach your goals.

To your health!

Philip J. Hoffman M.S., MBA

Body Transformation Coach

Fit-Lifestyle Model

Author

P.S. I'd love to see your testimonials! Please send them to:
phil@hoffmanfit.com

If you use Facebook, please like our page at:
http://www.facebook.com/hoffmanfit

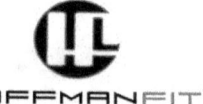

PERSONAL FITNESS TRAINING & NUTRITION CONSULTING

Master Grocery List

	Need?	Quantity		Need?	Quantity
Complex carbs: Fibrous			**Dairy**		
Asparagus			*Almond or coconut milk		
*Broccoli			*Low-fat cottage cheese		
Beets			*Eggs		
*Brussels sprouts			*Low-fat Greek yogurt		
Bell peppers			*Egg whites		
*Cabbage — red/green			**Proteins**		
Carrot			*Lean beef (organic grass fed)		
*Cauliflower			*Chicken		
Cucumber			*Pork-lean cuts		
Kale			*Fish: salmon, halibut, trout, tilapia		
*Lettuce – red leaf/romaine					
*Mushrooms					

*Onions, shallots, leeks					
Spinach					
*Tomatoes — fresh			**Sauces/Condiments & Spices/herbs**		
Turnips			*Balsamic vinegar		
Bok Choy			Ketchup/mustard		
Peeled tomatoes — canned			*Salsa, hot sauce		
Green beans			*Garlic cloves		
Peas			Ginger root		
			*Cinnamon		
Zucchini					
			Turmeric		
			Rosemary		
			Mint leaves		
			Simple Carbs : Fruits		
			Apples		
			Blueberries		
			Bananas		
			Cantaloupe/melons		
			Grapefruit		
Complex carbs: Starchy			Peaches		
Yams/ sweet potatoes			Pears		
Potatoes			Strawberries		
Beans			Papaya		
Lentils			Plums		
Brown rice			Cherries		
Oatmeal-steel cut			Grapes		
Squash			Kiwi		
Corn			Lemons/limes		
Quinoa			Oranges		

			Fats		
			*Flaxseed		
			Almonds		
			Walnuts		
			Pecans		
			Almond butter		
			*Avocado		
			Butter		

* Indicates a "core" item used for many of the essential meals in the *HoffmanFit System*

Appendix B

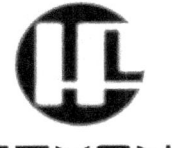

HOFFMANFIT
PERSONAL FITNESS TRAINING & NUTRITION CONSULTING

Daily Meal Log – Day 1

Name:

Date:

Meal	Food	Quantity (gms)	Protein (gms)	Carbs (gms)	Fat (gms)	Total Cal.
Breakfast	Egg (large)	1	6	0	5	72
	Egg whites	3	12	0	0	51
	Sweet potato protein pancake	1	16	9	2	120
	Coffee	Cup	0	0	0	0
	Half & half creamer	2 tbsp.	1	2	3	40
	Stevia natural sweetener	1 packet	0	0	0	0

Lunch	Salad/lettuce (any type, preferably dark green)	2 cups	2	3	0	20
	Sliced tomato	1 med	1	5	0	22
	Dressing (low-cal, any brand preferred)	4 tbsp.	2	4	7	90
	Pork tenderloin	4 oz.	32	0	5	185
Dinner	Turkey burger (extra lean)	8 oz.	46	0	4	240
	Cheese (slice of any type)	19 gm	4	1	3	45
	Avocado (medium)	1/2	1	3	13	125
	Ketchup (Heinz)	2 tbsp.	0	10	0	40
	Mustard (French's yellow classic)	1 tbsp.	0	0	0	0
	Mixed green salad & sliced tomato	2 cups	3	8	0	44
	Dressing	4 tbsp.	2	4	7	90
Snack	Protein shake (see breakfast recipes for macros)	Small	25	15	2	200
	Protein pancake	1	16	9	2	120
	Almond butter	2 tbsp.	8	8	16	190

Comments

Macronutrient totals: **Macronutrient ratios:**
Calories-1710   Protein-43%
Protein-177   Carbs-20%
Carbs-81   Fat-37%
Fat-69

HOFFMANFIT

PERSONAL FITNESS TRAINING & NUTRITION CONSULTING

Daily Meal Log – Day 2

Name:

Date:

Meal	Food	Quantity (gms)	Protein (gms)	Carbs (gms)	Fat (gms)	Total Cal.
Breakfast	Protein berry shake (see recipes for ingredients)	1	30	40	7	375
	Coffee & creamer (half & half)	2 tbsp.	1	2	3	40
Lunch	Protein pancake	1	16	9	2	120
	Scrambled eggs	2 large	12	0	5	144

Dinner	Large mixed green salad	3 cups	3	4.5	0	30
	Cherry tomatoes	5	1	6	0	28
	Broccoli florets	1 cup	3	4	0	25
	Salmon (broiled)	6 oz.	33	0	10	240
	Dressing (lite-any flavor)	3 tbsp.	0	10	6	105
Snack	Greek yogurt (plain, non-fat)	1 cup	22	7	0	120
	Protein powder (mix in yogurt)	½ scoop	15	0	2.5	65
	Crushed pecans (add to yogurt)	2 tbsp.	1	1	7	70
	Peanut butter	2 tbsp.	7	8	16	190
	Albacore tuna	can	24	0	1	100
	Dressing (lite-any flavor)	2 tbsp.	0	6	4	70

Comments

Macronutrient totals:
Calories-1722
Protein-165 gms
Carbs-97 gms
Fat-68 gms

Macronutrient ratios:
Protein-39%
Carbs-25%
Fat-36%

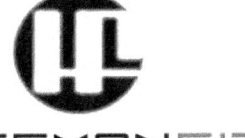

HOFFMANFIT

PERSONAL FITNESS TRAINING & NUTRITION CONSULTING

Daily Meal Log – Day 3

Name:

Date:

Meal	Food	Quantity (gms)	Protein (gms)	Carbs (gms)	Fat (gms)	Total Cal.
Breakfast	Coffee & cream (half & half)	2 tbsp.	1	2	3	40
	Steel cut oatmeal	¼ cup	5	27	0	150
	Protein powder (vanilla-Body Fortress brand)	½ scoop	15	0	1	65
	Blueberries or strawberries	½ cup	0	12	0	60
	Stevia natural sweetener	Packet	0	0	0	0
Lunch	Boneless pork chop (no fat)	4 oz.	30	0	2	140
	Greek yogurt	¾ cup	15	0	2	90
	Cucumber & tomato (mix in yogurt)	½ each	0	4	0	20

	Mixed green salad	Cup	0	2	0	20
	Dressing	2 tbsp.	1	4	2.5	45
Dinner	Chicken breast (grilled in skillet w/olive spray)	6 oz.	36	0	3	165
	Marinara sauce (see recipes to prepare)	½ cup	0	2	1	20
	Cauliflower (steamed)	Cup	2	5	0	25
	Parmesan cheese (grated)	2 tbsp.	1	1	2	20
	Green salad	3 cups	3	4.5	0	30
	Dressing (Lite-any flavor)	3 tbsp.	0	10	6	105
Snack	Protein pancake	1	16	9	2	120
	Almond butter (spread over pancake rolled up)	2 tbsp.	7	8	16	190
	Protein shake (lite version)	Small	25	15	2	200
	(see recipe for breakdown ingredients in shake)					

Comments

Macronutrient totals:
Calories-1505
Protein- 157gms
Carbs- 106 gms
Fat-41 gms

Macronutrient ratios:
Protein-43%
Carbs-32%
Fat-25%

HOFFMANꟻIT

PERSONAL FITNESS TRAINING & NUTRITION CONSULTING

Daily Meal Log – Day 4

Name:

Date:

Meal	Food	Quantity (gms)	Protein (gms)	Carbs (gms)	Fat (gms)	Total Cal.
Breakfast	Coffee & creamer (half & half)	2 tbsp.	1	2	3	40
	Protein pancake	1	16	9	2	120
	Scrambled egg whites	3	10	0	0	45
	Tomato & mushroom (sautéed in skillet)	Cup	1	2	0	15
	Cheese (any type)	1 oz.	4	1	3	45
Lunch	Green salad	3 cups	3	4.5	0	30
	Chicken breast (grilled, chopped into salad)	6 oz.	36	0	3	165
	Cherry tomatoes	5	1	6	0	28
	Broccoli (raw or steamed)	½ cup	2	2	0	15

	Dressing (lite-Paul Newman's honey mustard)	3 tbsp.	0	10	6	105
	Avocado (sliced into salad)	½ med.	1	3	13	125
Dinner	Tenderloin steak	4 oz.	32	0	8	203
	Asparagus (grilled in skillet or steamed)	8-10	2	4	0	20
	Mashed cauliflower (see recipe for ingredients)	Cup	8	12	1	80
	Green salad & sliced tomato	2 cups	2	3	0	20
	Dressing	2 tbsp.	1	4	2.5	45
	Grilled mushrooms (sautéed in skillet)	½ cup	1	1	0	10
	*use olive oil or coconut spray when cooking					
Snacks	Greek yogurt	Cup	22	7	0	120
	½ scoop chocolate protein powder (mix yogurt)	½	15	0	2.5	65
	Crushed pecans (add to yogurt to make dessert)	2 tbsp.	1	1	7	70
	Cottage cheese (lowfat 2%)	½ cup	11	6	2.5	90
	Cinnamon & Stevia sweetener	Packet	0	0	0	0
	Baked apple (chopped, add to cottage cheese)	1/2 cup	0	8	0	35

Comments	Macronutrient totals: ratios:	Macronutrient
	Calories-1631 Protein-170 gms Carbs-85 gms Fat-53 gms	Protein-44% Carbs-25% Fat-31%

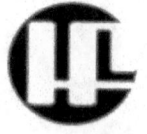

HOFFMANFIT

PERSONAL FITNESS TRAINING & NUTRITION CONSULTING

Daily Meal Log – Day 5

Name:

Date:

Meal	Food	Quantity (gms)	Protein (gms)	Carbs (gms)	Fat (gms)	Total Cal.
Breakfast	Coffee & creamer (half & half)		1	2	3	40
	Steel cut oatmeal	1/4 cup	5	27	0	150
	Protein powder (vanilla-Body Fortress brand)	½ scoop	15	0	1	65
	Blueberries or strawberries (any berry)	½ cup	0	12	0	60
	Stevia natural sweetener	packet	0	0	0	0
Lunch	Pita pocket Tuna salad (see recipes for totals)	Serving	28	36	3	300
	Cucumber & tomato salad (1/2 cuc,1/2 tom)	Serving	2	4	0	25

Dinner	Balsamic vinegar or lemon juice		0	0	0	0
	Italian spaghetti squash w/marinara &chicken	Serving	32	17	11	320
	(see recipes for breakdown ingredients)					
	(serving size accounts for all ingredients)					
	Green salad	3 cups	3	4.5	0	30
	Tomato, broccoli, mushrooms	2 cups	2	5	0	30
	Dressing (lite-any flavor)	3 tbsp.	0	10	6	105
Snack	Strawberry Protein Parfait dessert (recipe)	Serving	37	13	0	210
	Chicken breast	4 oz.	27	0	1	130
	Marinara sauce (pour over chicken)	½ Cup	0	2	1	20
	Parmesan or Romano cheese (sprinkle on sauce)	2 tbsp.	1	1	2	20

Comments

Macronutrient totals:
Calories-1495
Protein-152 gms
Carbs-143 gms
Fat-28 gms

Macronutrient ratios:
Protein-42%
Carbs-40%
Fat-18%

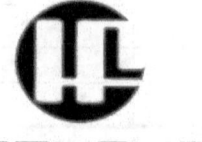

HOFFMANFIT

PERSONAL FITNESS TRAINING & NUTRITION CONSULTING

Daily Meal Log – Day 6

Name:

Date:

Meal	Food	Quantity (gms)	Protein (gms)	Carbs (gms)	Fat (gms)	Total Cal.
Breakfast	Coffee & creamer (half & half)	2 tbsp.	1	2	3	40
	Protein pancake	1	16	9	2	120
	Egg whites	3	10	0	0	45
Lunch	Green salad & tomato	3 cups	3	4.5	0	30
	Shredded pork tenderloin (see recipe on prep)	8 oz.	46	0	6	240
	Greek yogurt w/tomato, cucumber	½ cup	11	4	0	60
	(top pork with yogurt, squeezed lemon)					

132

Dinner	Chicken breast	6 oz.	36	0	3	165
	Baked yam or sweet potato	½ med.	1	20	0	90
	Broccoli (steamed)	Cup	2	2	0	15
Snack	Protein pancake	1	10	9	2	120
	Cinnamon apple yogurt (dessert)	Serving	31	8	0	210
	Almond butter	1 tbsp.	8	8	16	190
	Cottage cheese w/stevia sweetener	½ cup	11	6	2.5	90

Comments	**Macronutrient totals:** Calories-1415 Protein-180 gms Carbs-73 gms Fat-40 gms	**Macronutrient ratios:** Protein-50% Carbs-25% Fat-25%

133

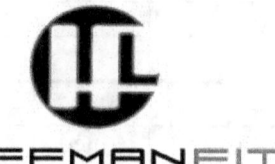

HOFFMANFIT

PERSONAL FITNESS TRAINING & NUTRITION CONSULTING

Daily Meal Log – Day 7

Name:

Date:

Meal	Food	Quantity (gms)	Protein (gms)	Carbs (gms)	Fat (gms)	Total Cal.
Breakfast	Coffee & creamer	2 tbsp	1	2	3	40
	Spinach & egg white scramble	4	13	0	0	60
	Cheese (any type)	1 oz.	4	1	3	45
	Broccoli & mushrooms (sautéed in skillet)	Cup	2	2	0	20
	Steal cut oatmeal	¼ cup	5	27	0	150
	Stevia sweetener	Packet				0
Lunch	Tropical chicken salad	Serving	57	30	10	400
	(see recipes for ingredients)					
	Cinnamon apple yogurt (see dessert recipes)	Serving	31	8	0	210

Dinner	Chicken stir fry (see recipes on preparing)	Serving	34	13	9	225
	Green salad w/tomato	3 cups	3	6	0	45
	Dressing (lite-any flavor)	3 tbsp.	0	10	6	105
Snack	Berry protein shake (see recipes on prep)	Serving	3	40	7	375
	Protein pancake	1	16	9	2	120
	Cottage cheese (roll up in pancake burrito style)	¼ cup	5	3	2	45
	Stevia sweetener (on cottage cheese)	Packet				0

Comments

Macronutrient totals:
Calories-1890
Protein- 174
Carbs- 152
Fat-41

Macronutrient ratios:
Protein-40%
Carbs-35%
Fat-25%

Appendix C – Recipes

~ **Breakfast Menu** ~

Protein Berry Shake

Ingredients:

Macronutrients per serving

- ¾ cup frozen strawberries
- ¾ cup frozen blueberries
- Whey isolate protein powder
- Ground flax seed, 1 tbsp.
- Cup Almond or coconut milk (low fat, sugar-free)

Calories: 280
Protein: 30g
Carbs: 32g
Fat: 2g

Directions:

- Place all ingredients in blender. Blend on high speed until smooth.

3:1 Egg White Omelet

Ingredients:

Macronutrients per serving

- 3 whites + 1 whole egg
- ¼ cup sliced mushrooms (optional)
- ¼ cup grated cheese (any variety)
- ¼ cup salsa

Calories: 210
Protein: 24g
Carbs: 10g
Fat: 8g

*Any vegetable item can be added

Directions:

- Have ingredients chopped and ready to add, along with eggs beaten
- Heat skillet over medium heat and spray with olive or coconut oil

- Pour eggs into skillet and let cook until edges around pan start to harden. Use spatula to spread uncooked portion of egg outward to corners so everything becomes cooked.
- When only small uncooked egg remains, add fillings of your choice to center of omelet.
- Fold one half of the omelet over the other and apply light pressure on top with your spatula.
- Remove omelet and serve.

Tip: This is a great breakfast for those that enjoy something more substantial in the morning. It's low in carbs and high in protein. Feel free to add or remove any of the above items. Any other vegetable can be added to this dish as well. You can also make a "3:1 easy scramble". Same ingredients are used so the calories and macronutrients don't change. It's also an easier and quicker method of preparation.

Sweet Potato Protein Pancakes

Ingredients: **Macronutrients per serving**

- 1 medium yam or sweet potato
- Scoop of vanilla whey isolate protein powder
- 1 tsp. baking powder
- 1 tsp. ground cinnamon
- ¾ cup egg white
- Coconut oil spray
(Makes 3- 4 pancakes; serving is one pancake)

Calories: 120
Protein: 16g
Carbs: 9g
Fat: 2g

Directions:

- Microwave the yam or sweet potato for approximately 7-8 minutes. Remove and let cool for about 10 minutes.
- Slice the yam long way and open so you can scoop out the meat with a spoon onto a plate and mash so it will be easier to mix in a bowl.

- In a medium-size mixing bowl, place the mashed yam and measure out ¾ cup egg whites, scoop of protein powder, tsp. baking powder and tsp. cinnamon and thoroughly whisk with an egg beater until batter is well mixed and appears like normal pancake batter. The yam should be well-broken up at this point.
- Heat a large skillet on medium heat and spray the pan with coconut oil. Using a large ladle, scoop enough batter to cover about 2/3 of the skillet. You don't want the batter to be too thick or the pancake takes too long to cook.
- Check after several minutes to see that the edges can be easily lifted and the pancake is dark brown in appearance. Then, quickly lift the pancake with one hand using a spatula and spray the pan right before flipping so the pancake won't stick. This is the tricky part.
- After the pancake is flipped, wait 30 sec or so and lightly tap down to flatten the pancake with your spatula to help cook the inside better. Remove when dark brown color. There should be enough batter to make between 3-4 pancakes. There are more than six ways to serve these pancakes with various toppings.

Steel-Cut Oats with Berries

Ingredients: **Macronutrients per serving**

- ⅓ cup steel-cut oatmeal (quick cook)
- Scoop vanilla whey protein powder
- ½ cup sliced berries (any type)
- 1 tsp. ground flax seed
- Stevia natural sweetener

Calories: 360
Protein: 37g
Carbs: 41g
Fat: 5g

Directions:

- Cook in microwave or stove top.

Italian Spaghetti Squash with Chicken Breast in Marinara Sauce

Ingredients:

Macronutrients per serving

- Spaghetti squash (medium, 3 lbs.)
- Peeled canned Italian tomatoes
- 1 lb. of chicken breast filets or tenders
- ¼ cup Romano grated cheese (or parmesan)
- Olive oil
- Two garlic cloves
- Black olives (optional)
- Tabasco sauce (optional) (Serves 4)

Calories: 320
Protein: 32g
Carbs: 17g
Fat: 11g

Directions:

How to cook spaghetti squash

- First cut it in half. Use a big knife, stab through the middle and wedge it down toward the outside. Then take out the knife and repeat on the other side working outwards. (It's easier than trying to cut through the whole thing at once).
- Scoop out the seeds and pulp in the cavity, and bake it in a 375 degree oven – face up – for about an hour – or until it looks like it's starting to dry out and you can easily insert a fork into the flesh.
- Lastly, when it's cooled down, take a fork and scrape out the strands. The more you separate them, the more volume you'll get! Store in fridge for up to four days to eat additional meals.

How to make marinara sauce

- Take a saucepan and place two minced garlic cloves with two tbsp. of olive oil and lightly sauté. Open the can of peeled tomatoes and break apart tomatoes with hands, removing any hard core pieces from the ends of tomatoes. Cento is the best brand peeled tomatoes.
- Add Tabasco and salt to your liking and let cook on low heat for 15 min. Add a dozen black olives sliced in half if desire.

Directions for serving:

- Using tongs, place the strands of spaghetti squash into a pasta bowl just as you would pasta. Generously spread the marinara sauce over the strands of squash and sprinkle with grated Romano or parmesan cheese while the sauce is still hot.
- The chicken breast can either be left as a larger piece on the side of the bowl, or you can slice and spread on top of the squash.

Boneless Chuck Roast in Slow Cooker

Ingredients:

Macronutrients per serving

- 1.5 lbs. boneless chuck roast
- 1 lb. raw carrots
- 1 large onion
- 2 oz. Worcestershire sauce

Calories: 383
Protein: 46g
Carbs: 11g
Fat: 14g

(Serves 4)

Prep time: 12 min

Directions:

- Place meat in the slow cooker.
- Peel onion and cut into wedges and place along sides of the roast.
- Cut ends of carrots off and wash before placing into slow cooker.

140

- Add 2 oz. of Worcestershire sauce along with enough water to cover the roast.
- Let it cook on high setting for at least six hours.
- There's almost no cleanup. Store the remaining portions for lunches or dinners during the week.

Tip: Using a slow cooker is one of the biggest time-savers you can use. You can turn the slow cooker on before going to bed and it will be cooked by morning, or you can safely let cook during the day while at work.

Pecan-Crusted Salmon with Mashed Cauliflower & Asparagus

Ingredients:

Macronutrients per serving

- 6 oz. Atlantic salmon
- 1 cup mashed cauliflower (already prepared)
- 8 spears of asparagus
- 1 tbsp. crushed pecans

Calories: 403
Protein: 40g
Carbs: 19g
Fat: 22g

Prep time: 10 min

Directions:

- Place crushed pecans on top of salmon fillet and broil in oven about 4 minutes each side.
- Steam asparagus in Zip N Steam bag in microwave.
- Squeeze juice of fresh lemon on salmon fillet and serve.

Boneless Pork Loin & Kale Salad

Ingredients: **Macronutrients per serving**

- 6 oz. boneless pork loin (trim any fat)   Calories: 438
- 1 cup chopped kale   Protein: 38g
  (see salad recipes for details)   Carbs: 17g
- 1 cooked yellow beet   Fat: 24g
- 2 tbsp. grated Romano cheese
- 2 tbsp. bread crumbs
- 1 tbsp. olive oil

Directions:

- Sear both sides of pork loin in a covered skillet until golden brown. Remove and serve.

Grass-Fed Beef Stir-Fry with Broccoli

Ingredients: **Macronutrients per serving**

- 2 teaspoons neutral-tasting oil,   Calories: 323
  such as canola or sunflower   Protein: 54g
- 3 garlic cloves, minced   Carbs: 4g
- pinch crushed red pepper flakes   Fat: 15g
- ½ pound boneless sirloin or tenderloin,
  cut into thin strips
- 1 ½ cups chopped broccoli
- 2 tbsp. low- sodium tamari soy sauce

(Serves 2)

Directions: Heat oil in a medium sauté pan over medium-high. Sauté garlic until just golden, stirring frequently, about 1 minute. Increase heat to high and add beef and broccoli. Cook until beef is seared and broccoli is crisp-tender, turning strips once, 2 to 3 minutes. Stir in tamari and serve immediately. You can add brown rice to this dish but keep portions small.

Spicy Broccoli with Chicken Breast & Fried Eggs

Ingredients: **Macronutrients per serving**

- 1 head broccoli, cut into florets
- 1 tbsp. olive oil, or olive oil spray
- 2 cloves garlic, thinly sliced
- ¼ tsp. red-pepper flakes
- ¼ lb. chicken breast
- salt and pepper to taste
- 2 eggs

Calories: 320
Protein: 30g
Carbs: 6g
Fat: 16g

Directions:

- Steam the broccoli in a Zip N Steam bag
- Heat the olive oil in a cast-iron skillet over medium heat. Add the garlic and red-pepper flakes and cook, stirring, for 1 minute. Add the chicken breast and broccoli and sauté until the chicken begins to brown. Season with salt and pepper and keep warm.
- In a separate skillet, fry the eggs sunny-side up in olive oil spray.

5-Minute Chicken Salad Sandwich

Ingredients: **Macronutrients per serving**

- 1 rib celery, finely chopped
- 1 tbsp. pine nuts
- 1 heaping tsp. spicy brown mustard
- 1 heaping tsp. fat-free sour cream
- 1 heaping tsp. plain non-fat yogurt
- pinch of ground black pepper
- 6 oz. of grilled chicken breast

Calories: 267
Protein: 28g
Carbs: 31g
Fat: 5g

- Thin Bun style bread (low carb)

(Serves 2)

Directions:

- In a large bowl, mix together the celery, pine nuts, mustard, sour cream, yogurt, and pepper. Add the chicken and toss lightly so you don't break apart too much.
- Divide the salad, spreading each half on a slice of thin bun bread.

Chili-Mango Chicken

Ingredients:	**Macronutrients per serving**

- 1 lb. boneless, skinless chicken breast cut into ½ -inch pieces
- 1 tbsp. cornstarch
- 1 tbsp. low-sodium soy sauce
- ½ tbsp. sesame oil
- ½ tbsp. peanut or canola oil
- 1 onion chopped
- 1 tbsp. grated or minced fresh ginger
- 2 cups sugar snap peas
- 1 mango, peeled, pitted and chopped
- 1 tbsp. chili garlic sauce (Huy Fong)
- Black pepper to taste
  (Serves 2)

Calories: 361
Protein: 31g
Carbs: 20g
Fat: 16g

Directions:

- Minutes 0-12: marinate the chicken. Combine the chicken pieces, cornstarch, soy sauce, and sesame oil in a mixing bowl, and let it sit for 10 minutes.

- Minutes 12-17: stir fry the vegetables on a wok or large skillet, heat the peanut or canola oil on high. Add the onion and ginger and cook until the onion is translucent, 1 to 2 minutes. Add the peas and stir fry for 1 minute.
- Minutes 17-19: Add the mango, chili garlic sauce, and pepper. Stir-fry until the chicken is cooked through and the mango becomes saucy, about 1 minute more. Serve over brown rice.

Tip: If sugar snaps are too pricey or hard to find, go with snow peas, green beans, or even broccoli florets.

Low Carb Chicken Taco Wraps

Ingredients:

Macronutrients per serving

Calories: 494
Protein: 50g
Carbs: 28g
Fat: 24g

- 6 oz. chicken breast
- Low-carb tortillas
- ½ avocado thinly sliced
- ½ medium tomato diced
- 2 tbsp. shredded cheddar cheese
- 2 tbsp. low-fat sour cream
- 2 tbsp. salsa
- Olive oil spray

(2 tacos = 1 serving)

Directions:

- Cut up chicken breast into small bite-size pieces in skillet and cook in olive oil spray.
- Take ½ romaine lettuce shell and place chicken and sample of each remaining ingredient on top of shell. Then cover the ingredients with another shell to make a closed wrap-like taco.

Tip: If you want to reduce your carb intake, find Romaine lettuce to use as wraps to replace the traditional flour tortillas.

Beef Tenderloin Steak Dinner

Ingredients: **Macronutrients per serving**

- 6 oz. organic grass-fed tenderloin
- 1 cup mixed green salad with tomato
  (See daily mixed green salad recipe)
- 1 cup mashed cauliflower (see recipe)

Calories: 571
Protein: 52g
Carbs: 27g
Fat: 21g

Directions:

- Grill or broil steak as desired and serve with mashed cauliflower.

Tip: This is a delicious meal for anyone wanting red meat without consuming a large quantity of calories.

Chicken Stir Fry

Ingredients: **Macronutrients per serving**

- 8 oz. chicken breast
- 1 cup vegetable stir fry package
- 1 tbsp. coconut oil (organic, virgin)
- 2 tbsp. hoisin sauce
- 2 tbsp. soy sauce

Calories: 225
Protein: 34g
Carbs: 13g
Fat: 8.5g

(Serves 2)

Directions:

- Cook chicken in a skillet with tbsp. coconut oil.

- Cook stir fry vegetables with hoisin sauce in a separate, deep skillet or wok on high heat until tender yet crisp. Add cooked chicken breast, mix thoroughly and serve.

**Add more broccoli, snow peas or carrots to increase the quantity of vegetables desired.

Trout (Rainbow or Steelhead) with Asparagus

Ingredients: **Macronutrients per serving**

- 6 oz. steelhead trout (rainbow trout)
- 8 medium spears asparagus
- 1 tbsp. olive oil
- 1 lemon, sliced

Calories: 366
Protein: 32g
Carbs: 5g
Fat: 25g

Directions:

- Place trout in small pan with sliced lemon and squeeze juice over fish.
- Bake at 400 degrees for about 12 minutes.
- Grill asparagus in skillet with 1 tbsp. olive oil until tender.

Tip: Trout is as good or better tasting a fish as salmon at half the price and also provides a good quantity of omega fatty acids.

Pita Pocket Tuna Salad

Ingredients: **Macronutrients per serving**

- Can albacore solid white tuna (4 oz.)
- 1 tbsp. raisins (or chopped prunes or dates)
- 2 tbsp. chopped celery
- ¼ cup chopped apple
- 2 tbsp. Veganaise (or other low cal product)

Calories: 299
Protein: 27g
Carbs: 41g
Fat: 4g

- 1 tsp. Dijon mustard
- ½ pita pocket (low-carb)

Directions:

- Place ingredients into a small mixing bowl and thoroughly mix.
- Fill both halves of pocket with salad and serve.

Tropical Chicken Salad

Ingredients: **Macronutrients per serving**

- 6 oz. boneless chicken breast
- 2 cups chopped romaine lettuce
- ½ cup plain non-fat Greek yogurt
- ¼ cup chopped apple
- ¼ cup orange cut in small pieces
- 1 tbsp. chopped pecans
- ¼ cup grapes cut in half
- 2 tbsp. celery chopped
- Add seasoning as desired

Calories: 414
Protein: 57g
Carbs: 31g
Fat: 10g

Directions:

- Place all ingredients into small mixing bowl and thoroughly mix. Add salt and pepper as desired and serve.

Strawberry & Pecan Mixed-Green Salad with Chicken Breast

Ingredients:

Macronutrients per serving

- 2 cups mixed green salad (any variety)
- 6 cherry tomatoes
- 4 large strawberries (1 cup) sliced
- 1 tbsp. pecans crushed
- 1 tbsp. olive oil
- ½ squeezed lemon
- 1 packet Stevia natural sweetener
- 6 oz. grilled chicken breast

Calories: 495
Protein: 56g
Carbs: 28g
Fat: 24g

Directions:

- In a small bowl, pour squeezed lemon, olive oil and Stevia and mix. Place salad and remaining ingredients in a large salad bowl and pour dressing over salad.
- Top salad with grilled chicken breast

Baby Kale Salad with Salmon

Ingredients:

Macronutrients per serving

- 6 oz. salmon
- 1 cup pre-washed baby kale (any variety of greens)
- 1 cup cherry tomatoes, sliced
- 4 small broccoli florets
- 2 tbsp. olive oil

Calories: 560
Protein: 36g
Carbs: 20g
Fat: 38g

Directions:

- Broil salmon for 7 minutes each side. Break into small pieces and let cool.
- Place salad into large salad bowl and add sliced tomatoes, broccoli.

- Place the salmon pieces on top of the salad.
- Squeeze juice of lemon into small bowl and mix with olive oil and then pour over salad and serve.

Thai Chicken Salad

Ingredients: **Macronutrients per serving**

- 6 oz. of chicken breast (cut 1" cubes)
- 1 cup mixed green salad (any variety)
- 1 cup cherry tomatoes (halved)
- 1 cup cabbage, chopped (green or red)
- ½ medium cucumber sliced
- 2 tbsp. Thai peanut dressing

Calories: 438
Protein: 54g
Carbs: 21g
Fat: 19g

Directions:

- Place all ingredients into a large salad bowl, including the chicken. Top with the Thai peanut dressing and thoroughly mix so the dressing covers the ingredients and serve.

Tip: Remember, the chicken breast used for this salad has already been cooked during one of your food prep sessions.

Whole Organic Chicken in Slow Cooker

Ingredients: **Macronutrients per serving**

- Organic chicken grill pack – includes 2 split breasts, 4 drumsticks
- 1 large onion, chopped
- 3 large tomatoes (cut into wedges)
- 2 garlic cloves

Calories: 196
Protein: 23g
Carbs: 7g
Fat: 9g

(Serves 4-6)

Directions:

- Place all ingredients into slow cooker and add spices, salt and pepper to your liking. Cover with water and let cook on low heat for approximately 8-10 hours, depending on the type of slow cooker.

Tip: You can cook before going to bed, or cook during the day while at work. Prep time is less than 10 minutes and you'll have an excellent source of protein that can be used for multiple types of meals. Cleanup is also minimal since everything is in one pot.

Organic Hawaiian Burger

Ingredients:	**Macronutrients per serving**

- 1/3 lb. Organic grass-fed ground beef
- ½ oz. Swiss cheese
- 1 pineapple slice
- ½ pita pocket bread
- Splash of teriyaki sauce

Calories: 497
Protein: 30.5g
Carbs: 27g
Fat: 23g

Direction:

- Grill 1/3 lb. of organic grass-fed beef patty, either on an outdoor grill or stove to make three burgers
- Place cheese on burger so that it melts
- Add pineapple and teriyaki sauce and place inside of pita pocket and serve

**Feel free to add any other topping like lettuce or mushrooms, or condiments like ketchup and mustard.

Homemade Italian Marinara Sauce

Ingredients: **Macronutrients per serving**

- 1 can Italian peeled tomatoes (Cento brand)   Calories: 55
- 2 cloves garlic crushed   Protein: 1g
- 12 black or Kalamata pitted olives (halved)   Carbs: 4g
- 1 tbsp. olive oil   Fat: 4g
- Tabasco sauce (optional)

(Makes about 4 servings)

Directions:

- In a sauce pan, pour olive oil and garlic cloves and sauté for a couple minutes on low heat.
- Open can of peeled tomatoes and break apart into small pieces into a medium bowl. Then pour the tomatoes in the sauce pan and let it cook on medium heat for 5-10 minutes.
- Add Tabasco sauce if you prefer spicy sauce.
- Store sauce in a container in the refrigerator to use throughout the week for many other dishes.

3-Veggie Chicken Salad

Ingredients: **Macronutrients per serving**

- 6 oz. grilled chicken breast   Calories: 288
- 1 cup red cabbage, chopped   Protein: 36g
- 1 cup broccoli florets, chopped   Carbs: 19g
- 6 cherry tomatoes   Fat: 7g
- 2 tbsp. dressing (any type of low-cal)

Directions:

- Place all ingredients into salad bowl. Cut chicken breast into strips. Top with dressing and mix.

152

Tip: All ingredients for salads like this have been prepared during one of your food prep sessions.

Seared Ahi Tuna with Cabbage Slaw

Ingredients:

Macronutrients per serving

- 6 oz. ahi tuna steak
- ½ cup red or green cabbage
- ½ cup shredded carrots
- 1 tbsp. sesame oil
- 2 tbsp. tamari or soy sauce
- 1 tbsp. ginger, freshly ground
- 1 clove garlic, minced
- 1 tsp. lime juice

Calories: 355
Protein: 42g
Carbs: 7g
Fat: 15.5g

Directions:

- Mix marinade ingredients together and coat tuna steak, cover and let sit in refrigerator for at least an hour.
- Heat non-stick skillet over medium to high heat. Remove tuna steak from marinade and sear for two minutes each side. If you prefer more well-done, sear for 2.5 minutes each side.
- Remove from skillet and serve with cabbage slaw.

Spicy Buffalo Chicken Tenders

Ingredients:

Macronutrients per serving

- 6 oz. chicken tenders
- 2 tbsp. ranch dressing (lite)
- 4 tbsp. spicy wing sauce
- Olive oil spray

Calories: 260
Protein: 50g
Carbs: 7g
Fat: 5g

Directions:

- Grill chicken tenders in skillet on stove-top. Remove and prepare spicy sauce mix for dipping.

Tip: Mix sauce according to how spicy you prefer your dip. This is a very high-protein, low-carb dish to accompany a salad.

Batch-Cooking of Protein Sources for Storage

Preparing protein sources in advance and having for quick serving is essential for busy people that don't have time to prepare single meals. You can use the various protein sources throughout the week.

Here are some examples of how to prepare protein sources:

Preparation of chicken breast using a slow-cooker or crock-pot

Directions:

- Prepare desired quantity of chicken you want according to number of family members. If you plan on freezing most of it, then make sure to cook at least 4 lbs. of chicken breasts.
- You can also cook an entire chicken, but it's much easier and cleaner to cook breast meat without bones or skin. It also makes for minimal clean-up.
- Add spices and condiments desired like salt, pepper, lemon pepper, garlic or onion. Top chicken breast with water until meat is covered.
- Depending on the style and model of slow cooker you have, cook for about 4-8 hours.
- Sample the meat at various times so you know how fast your slow cooker cooks the chicken.

- When cooked, remove chicken and place into either Tupperware containers or freezer bags with portioned amount of chicken for freezing. For example, I prefer to weigh out 12 oz. servings into baggies and freeze. Each baggie provides two 6 oz. servings for meals.
- Cleanup of the slow cooker is less than 5 minutes. It's by far the fastest method I've found for making my chicken for everyday salads, or a variety of other meals that chicken is used.

Preparation of grilled chicken tenders

- If you'd like to add another method of preparing chicken, you can grill and store for freezing the same way you did using the slow cooker.
- The only difference is you will now grill the chicken tenders either in a skillet on your stove-top or your outdoor grill.
- Be careful not to overcook so that chicken becomes dry.
- Store portions for freezing according to number of family members.

Preparation of baked chicken breast in oven

- Baking chicken breast on a large oven pan is also quick and easy. Preferably use larger chicken breasts instead of tenders for baking so they don't become too dried out. Bake for about 30 minutes and flip to cook another 15 minutes, depending on the thickness of the breasts.
- Let cook and wrap in a piece of wax paper and place each individual breast into a storage bag for quick removal from the freezer.

Preparation of fish such as salmon and trout

- Fish cannot be cooked in advance and stored or frozen. Instead, what you can do is purchase larger quantities of salmon and cut into 6 oz. portions and freeze for quick removal. For example, if you plan on making salmon for dinner, remove a portioned piece from the freezer in the morning before work so it's ready to cook in the evening.
- Weigh your protein sources for accurately measuring calorie and nutrient intake

~ Vegetable Side Dishes ~

Mashed Cauliflower (use in place of mashed potatoes)

Ingredients: **Macronutrients per serving**

- Large head of cauliflower
  (or package of florets)
- ½ cup plain non-fat Greek yogurt
- ¼ cup grated Romano or parmesan cheese

Calories: 80
Protein: 7.5g
Carbs: 12g
Fat: 1g

(Serves 4)

Directions:

- How to cut cauliflower: Remove the leaves from the cauliflower. Cut around the underside of the head, removing most of the core. Detach the florets where they join at the center. Separate the florets by cutting through the base to make smaller florets. Cut any size floret you like by simply cutting through stem and head of each floret.
- Fill Ziploc Zip'n Steam bags with cauliflower and steam in microwave for 5 minutes each bag or steam on stove top.
- Place steamed cauliflower in food processor with yogurt until creamy. Now place contents in a serving bowl and mix in grated cheese and salt and pepper as desired. You can also use an old-fashioned potato masher instead of a food processor to mash.

Tip: This side dish can be eaten with many protein dishes. For most people, the consistency and flavor is almost the same as mashed potatoes, yet has half the calories and is much higher in phytonutrients.

**You can prepare this side dish during one of your prep sessions and keep all week in the refrigerator without spoiling.

Chopped Brussels Sprouts With Sun-Dried Tomato

Ingredients: **Macronutrients per serving**

- Brussels sprouts (30 sprouts)
- ¼ cup sun-dried tomato in olive oil
- ¼ cup slivered almonds
- Fresh lemon

Calories: 170
Protein: 8g
Carbs: 8g
Fat: 19g

(Serves 4)

Directions:

- Steam Brussels sprouts either on a stove top or using Zip N Steam bag in the microwave. Stove top takes about 12 minutes. Place in fridge or freezer to cool for 10 minutes.
- Chop sprouts on a cutting board and throw into mixing bowl. Squeeze lemon and toss.
- Serve in bowl and sprinkle desired amount of sun-dried tomato and slivered almonds.

Tip: No need to add extra olive oil because the sun-dried tomatoes are already coated.

Broccoli Slaw

Ingredients: **Macronutrients per serving**

- 4 cups broccoli
- 4 cups red cabbage
- 4 oz. Greek honey yogurt

Calories: 90
Protein: 4g
Carbs: 13g
Fat: 2g

(Serves 4)

Directions:

- Wash broccoli and cut up florets before placing in food processor.
- Finely slice red cabbage on cutting board.

- Fill food processor and quickly chop so broccoli and cabbage are in small pieces but not minced. Toss chopped pieces into mixing bowl and place remaining pieces into food processor until all chopped.
- Place 4 oz. of Greek honey yogurt into mixing bowl with chopped broccoli and cabbage and thoroughly mix until yogurt has coated everything.
- Chill in fridge for 10 minutes and serve.

Tip: Nowadays, there are many brands of pre-washed and sliced vegetable combinations/mixtures similar to this. If you prefer to save more time, you can go this route.

3-C salad (cabbage, carrot, cucumber)

Ingredients: **Macronutrients per serving**

- 1 cup cabbage chopped (green or red)
- ½ cup shredded carrots
- 1 cup cucumbers, sliced
- 6 cherry tomatoes, halved
- 2 tbsp. any low-cal dressing

Calories: 166
Protein: 4g
Carbs: 29g
Fat: 4g

Directions:

- In a medium size mixing bowl, combine ingredients and add dressing.
- Thoroughly mix and serve.

Tip: If you want to make this a protein-packed meal, add 4-6 oz. of chicken breast

Mixed Green Salad & Tomato

Ingredients: **Macronutrients per serving**

- 2 cups mixed green salad
  (any variety, including spinach)
- 1 medium tomato or 6 cherry tomatoes
- 2 tbsp. low-cal dressing
- Squeezed lemon or balsamic vinegar
- Salt and pepper

Calories: 111
Protein: 3g
Carbs: 15g
Fat: 4g

Directions:

- Fill a large serving bowl with 2-3 cups of any variety of dark green lettuce or spinach. Add tomato and dressing or balsamic vinegar and toss. Add salt and pepper as desired and serve.

Tip: Find a salad that you enjoy eating and prepare it daily. It should be a staple in the diet. You can add any variety of vegetable to this salad and eat unlimited quantities without concern. Just for an example, the lettuce in this salad only has 23 calories. It could be disregarded as far as calories are concerned.

**If you have a special dressing that you prefer to replace the olive oil and lemon or vinegar, you can do so as long as you measure with a tablespoon so you know exactly how much is used. Many people easily consume over 400 calories of dressing without knowing.

Strawberry-Pecan Mixed-Green Salad (see previous version which includes chicken)

Ingredients: **Macronutrients per serving**

- 2 cups mixed green salad (any variety)
- 1 Medium tomato or 6 cherry tomatoes

Calories: 352
Protein: 7g
Carbs: 32g
Fat: 23g

- 4 large strawberries (1 cup) sliced
- 1 tbsp. pecans crushed
- 2 tbsp. low-cal dressing

Directions:

- In a small bowl, pour squeezed lemon, dressing and mix. Place salad and remaining ingredients in a large salad bowl and pour dressing over salad and serve.

Tuscan Kale Salad

Ingredients:	Macronutrients per serving

- 2 cups pre-washed organic baby kale
- 2 tbsp. olive oil
- ½ cup grated parmesan cheese
- Fresh squeezed lemon
- Salt & pepper

Calories: 275
Protein: 7g
Carbs: 9g
Fat: 25g

Directions:

- Place 2 cups of kale in a large bowl.
- Mix together in a small mixing bowl the lemon juice, olive oil, salt and pepper.
- Pour over the kale and toss well.
- Add the grated cheese and toss again before serving.

Greek Banana Protein Pudding

Ingredients: **Macronutrients per serving**

- ¾ cup plain non-fat Greek yogurt
- ½ scoop vanilla whey isolate
  protein powder
- ½ sliced medium banana
- 1 packet Stevia natural sweetener

Calories: 200
Protein: 29g
Carbs: 18g
Fat: 0g

Directions:

- Slice banana and place all ingredients into small mixing bowl and thoroughly mix together and serve.

Tip: This is a great snack when you have a craving for something sweet. It also works well for an on-the-go breakfast because you can prepare it the night before.

Cottage Cheese with Baked Cinnamon Apple

Ingredients: **Macronutrients per serving**

- ½ cup low fat cottage cheese
- ½ medium apple
- Dash of cinnamon
- Packet of Stevia sweetener

Calories: 130
Protein: 11g
Carbs: 17g
Fat: 2g

Directions:

- Cut the apple into quarters for easier removal of the skin and core. Using half the apple, chop the pieces into smaller chunks and microwave in a small bowl for up to 90 seconds.
- Scoop eight ounces of cottage cheese into a bowl with the warm apple before sprinkling in cinnamon and your packet of Stevia natural sweetener. Thoroughly mix and serve.

Cinnamon Apple Yogurt

Ingredients: **Macronutrients per serving**

- ¾ cup non-fat plain Greek yogurt
- ½ apple, peeled and chopped
- ½ scoop vanilla whey isolate protein powder
- 1 packet Stevia natural sweetener
- Pinch of cinnamon

Calories: 185
Protein: 29g
Carbs: 15g
Fat: 0g

Directions:

- Place ingredients into a small mixing bowl, thoroughly mix and serve.

Blueberry or Strawberry Protein Parfait

Ingredients: **Macronutrients per serving**

- ¾ cup plain non-fat Greek yogurt
- ½ scoop vanilla whey isolate protein powder
- ½ cup sliced strawberries (or blueberries)
- 1 packet Stevia natural sweetener

Calories: 170
Protein: 29g
Carbs: 10g
Fat: 0g

Directions:

- Place ingredients into small mixing bowl, thoroughly stir and serve.

Tip: This is another excellent low-calorie dessert. Finding a dessert or snack that provides as much satiety as this isn't easy. You can also add a sprinkle of pecans to give it even more flavor, but remember to consider the added calories.

Cottage Cheese Almond Butter Spread

Ingredients:	Macronutrients per serving
• ¾ cup low fat cottage cheese • 1 tbsp. almond butter • 1 packet Stevia natural sweetener	Calories: 235 Protein: 24g Carbs: 9.5g Fat: 11g

Directions:

- Place all ingredients in a small mixing bowl and thoroughly mix so the almond butter is mixed in well.

Tip: This is a great breakfast snack if you're in a hurry yet need something quick. It also makes for a great dip alternative on vegetables because of the high protein added from the cottage cheese.

Protein Pancake with Greek Yogurt & Pecans (burrito style)*

Ingredients: **Macronutrients per serving**

- Protein pancake   Calories: 200
- 1 tbsp. Greek yogurt   Protein: 17g
- 1 tbsp. Pecan pieces   Carbs: 9g
- 1 packet Stevia sweetener   Fat: 9g

Directions:

- Take one pancake and spread tablespoon of non-fat plain Greek yogurt down center of pancake.
- Sprinkle tablespoon of pecans on top of yogurt, sprinkle sweetener and roll into a burrito-style wrap.

Tip: This is a great on-the-run breakfast with coffee or late-night snack when you have a craving for something sweet.

**There are multiple ways to serve these delicious Protein Pancakes. Please refer to the *HoffmanFit* blog for more ideas.

Chocolate Protein Yogurt with Pecans/Walnuts

Ingredients: **Macronutrients per serving**

- 1 cup of plain low-fat yogurt   Calories: 263
- ½ scoop chocolate protein powder   Protein: 27g
- 1 tbsp. pecans or walnuts, crushed   Carbs: 20g
  (optional)   Fat: 7g
- 1 packet of Stevia natural sweetener
  (optional)

Directions:

- Place all ingredients into a serving bowl, thoroughly mix and serve.

Exercises

Legs: quadriceps, hamstrings, glutes

1. Dumbbell squats

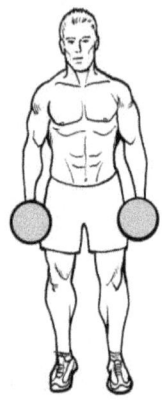 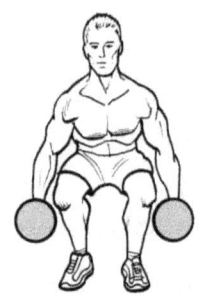

Starting position: Hold two dumbbells at your sides, with your palms facing in. Stand with your feet about shoulder width apart. If you have trouble balancing, try placing a couple of dumbbell plates under your heels.

The exercise: While keeping your shoulders back and head upright, bend your legs at the knees and lower your hips until your thighs are parallel with the floor. Then, pushing from your heels, lift yourself back up to the starting position. Keep your back as straight as possible throughout this exercise.

Muscles worked:

Primary: quadriceps, hamstrings, gluteal

Secondary: erector spinae, abs, hip flexors

2. Romanian deadlifts

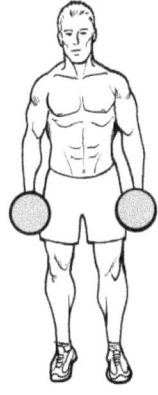 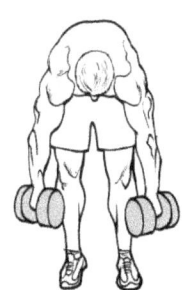

Starting position: Stand up straight, with your feet shoulder width apart and a dumbbell in each hand, your palms facing toward your legs. This is a great exercise for the hamstrings, and it helps strengthen the lower back.

The exercise: Bend forward at your hips, and slowly lower the dumbbells in front of you until the weights almost touch the floor. Keep your back straight throughout the exercise. Then, while concentrating on the muscles in the back of your legs, raise your upper body and the weights to the starting position.

Tip: Don't hunch over. Keep your back flat throughout the exercise.

Muscles worked:

Primary: gluteal, hamstrings

Secondary: erector spinae, abs

3. Dumbbell lunges

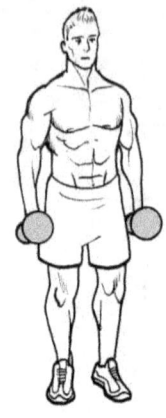 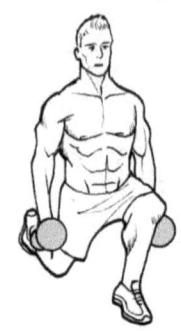

Starting position: Stand with your feet together, holding a dumbbell in each hand at your sides, palms facing in. Take a large step forward with your left leg. When your front thigh is parallel to the floor and your back knee is a few inches off the floor, hold for a second. Then return to starting position and repeat with your right leg.

Tip: Be sure to keep your knee from extending over your toes, which can cause injury. Lunges can be done without the weights if it's too difficult.

Muscles worked:

Primary: quadriceps, hamstrings, gluteal

Secondary: abs

4. Goblet squat

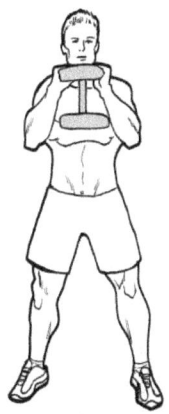 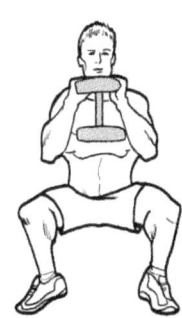

Starting position: Hold a dumbbell while cupping the top with feet about shoulder-width apart. Hold the weight close to your chest.

The exercise: Squat down, lowering your hips and glutes deep enough to feel a strong stretch in the entire leg. The elbows remain to the inside of the knees while performing the squat. Keep the torso upright and the abs engaged as you push with the heels of your feet.

Tip: Push from the heels of your feet rather than the front of your foot to help maintain proper back position.

Muscles worked:

Primary: quadriceps, gluteal, hamstrings

Secondary: erector spinae, abs

5. Wide-grip pull downs

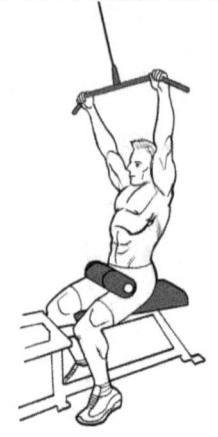 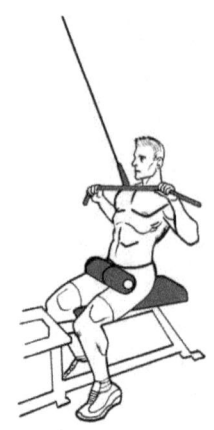

Starting position: Seated on a bench or pulldown machine, grasp a wide bar wider than shoulder width.

The exercise: Pull the bar down to the top of your chest. Focus on keeping your elbows directly below the bar. Arch your back slightly, and hold the bar in that position right on top of your collarbone for a second, then slowly let the bar back up to the starting position.

Tip: Don't lean back too far and pull the weight down using momentum.

Muscles worked:

Primary: latissimus dorsi, rhomboids, teres major

Secondary: trapezius, erector spinae

6. One-arm dumbbell row

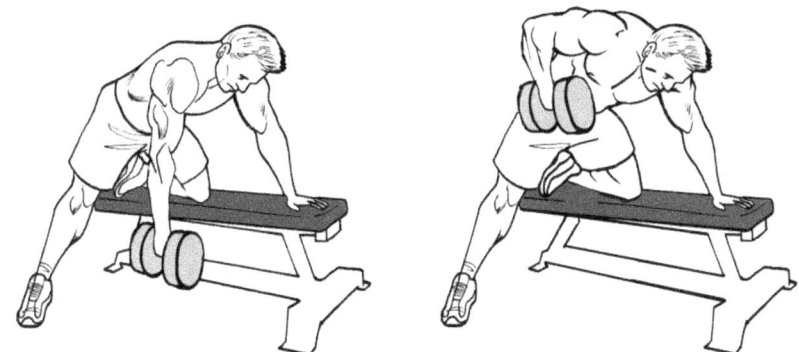

Starting position: Start with your right foot flat on the floor and your left knee resting on the bench. Then lean forward so you're supporting yourself with your left arm on the bench. Your back should be parallel to the floor. Reach down and grab the dumbbell with your right hand. Look straight ahead instead of at the floor so your back stays straight.

The exercise: Concentrate on pulling your elbow as far back as it can go. The dumbbell should end up roughly parallel with your torso. After you've rowed the dumbbell up as far as you can, slowly lower it to the starting position. After you complete the set of reps, switch to your right arm and do the same thing.

Tip: Don't hunch your back. Keep it flat and parallel to the floor.

Muscles worked:

Primary: latissimus dorsi, rhomboids, teres major

Secondary: trapezius, erector spinae

7. Assisted pull-ups (with band)

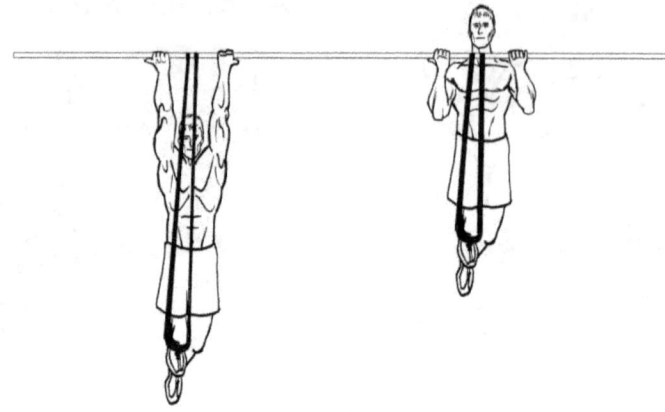

Starting position: Choke the band around the center of the pull up bar. You can use different bands to provide varying levels of assistance. Pull the end of the band down, and place one bent knee into the loop, ensuring it won't slip out. Take a medium to wide grip on the bar. This will be your starting position.

The exercise: Pull yourself upward by contracting the lats as you flex the elbow. Pull to the front, attempting to get your chin over the bar. Avoid swinging or jerking movements.

Tip: This exercise requires on-site demonstration to understand proper movement.

Muscles worked:

Primary: latissimus dorsi

Secondary: biceps, brachialis, brachioradialis, teres major and minor, posterior deltoid, trapezius, rhomboids, pectoralis minor, levator scapulae

Chest

8. Dumbbell bench press

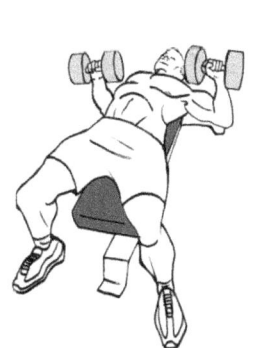 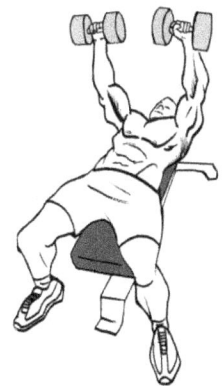

Starting position: Lie flat on a bench with feet flat on floor. Hold a dumbbell in each hand just above your shoulders, with your palms facing forward and your elbows out at sides.

The exercise: Press the weights up until the arms are fully extended and locked, then slowly lower the weights back to the sides of your chest.

Tip: The path of the weights should follow in a straight line over your collarbone, not your face or upper abdominal region.

Muscles worked:

Primary: pectoralis major and triceps brachii

Secondary: anterior and posterior deltoid

9. Incline dumbbell press

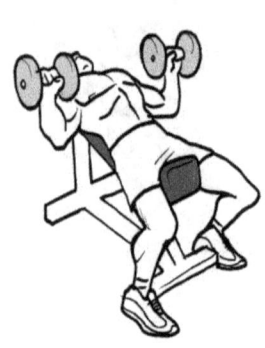 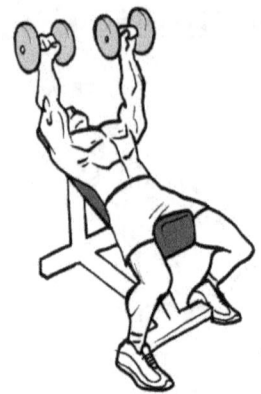

Starting position: Lie on an incline bench with feet flat on the floor. Hold a pair of dumbbells above your chest, arms extended using an overhand grip.

The exercise: Lower the dumbbells toward the sides of your chest, pause for a second, then forcefully push them back to the starting position.

Tip: The bench should not be inclined more than about 30 degrees for this exercise, otherwise there's too much shoulder involvement.

Muscles worked:

Primary: pectoralis major and minor

Secondary: anterior and posterior deltoids, triceps

Shoulder

10. Seated dumbbell press

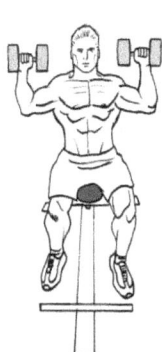 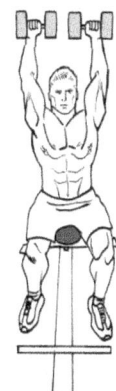

Starting position: Sit on a bench with feet flat on floor. Hold a dumbbell in each hand at shoulder height, elbows out and palms facing forward.

The exercise: Press the dumbbells up and together so they almost touch above your head. Don't allow the weights to stray back and forth. Press the weights up until your arms are almost fully extended straight. Then, slowly lower the dumbbells to the starting position.

Tip: Look straight forward with chin up, shoulders squared and chest high.

Muscles worked:

Primary: deltoids, trapezius

Secondary: triceps

11. Side DB raises

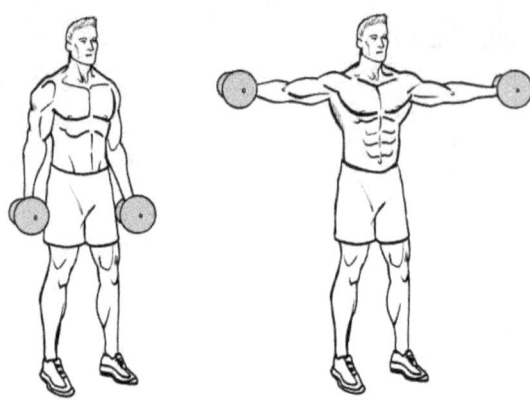

Starting position: Stand upright with your feet about shoulder width apart and your arms at your sides. Hold a dumbbell in each hand, your palms turned toward your body. Keep your palms turned downward as you lift the dumbbells so your shoulders, rather than your biceps, do the work.

The exercise: Keeping your arms straight, life the weights out and up to the sides until they are right about level with your chin, and hold them there for a second. From this position, lower them slowly back to your sides.

Tip: Don't lean back and swing the weights up. Lift them straight out to your sides until they're almost directly out from your shoulders. At the top position, it appears like a gymnast doing an iron cross on the rings. Don't lean forward and allow the dumbbells down in front of your body, either. Instead, let the weights down to your sides.

Muscles worked:

Primary: supraspinatus, lateral deltoid

Secondary: Trapezius, abs

12. Upright DB row

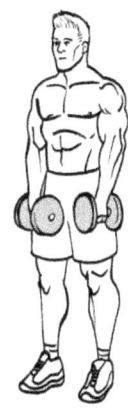 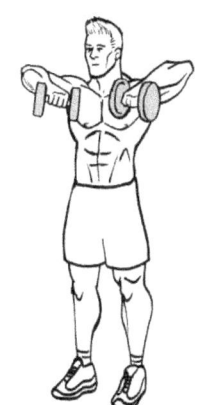

Starting position: Stand with a DB in each hand at the sides of your thighs with feet placed at shoulder width.

The exercise: Lift both dumbbells upward until your arms are slightly higher than parallel to the ground, or just under your chin. Then lower the weights down slowly after a short pause at the top.

Tip: Do not allow gravity to let the weights drop when lowering them. Also, concentrate on the lift initiated from the elbows to maintain proper form.

Muscles worked:

Primary: deltoids, trapezius

Triceps

13. Cable pressdowns

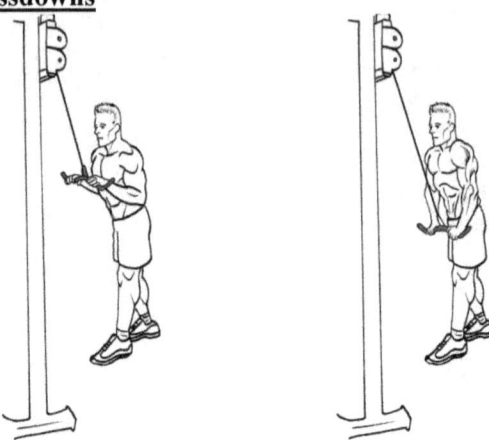

Starting position: Stand in front of the cable machine with feet shoulder width apart. Grab the bar with your hands about eight inches apart, palms facing downward.

The exercise: Push down the bar in an arc-like movement until the arms are extended and locked out. Pause for a second and follow the same arc movement back to the starting position. Always maintain tension on the triceps.

Tip: Keep your arms firmly positioned at your sides so your elbows don't flair outward during the movement.

Muscles worked:

Primary: triceps

Secondary: muscles of posterior forearm

14. Skull crushers (EZ-bar extension)

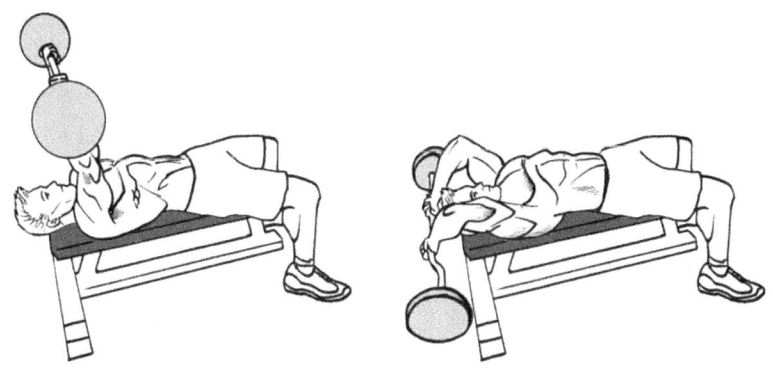

Starting position: Grab a barbell and lie down on a bench. Your hands should be about a foot apart on the bar. Press the bar up so your arms are extended straight and weight is over your upper chest/shoulder region.

The exercise: Lower the bar down to the top of the forehead while elbows remain stationary, pointing towards the ceiling. Now press the barbell back to the starting point using the same arc of motion.

Tip: Lower the bar slowly behind the head for a longer range of motion, keeping elbows locked in position to isolate the triceps. Using an E-Z curl bar vs. straight bar reduces pressure on the wrist joint.

Muscles worked:

Primary: triceps

Secondary: deltoids, abs

15. Bench dips

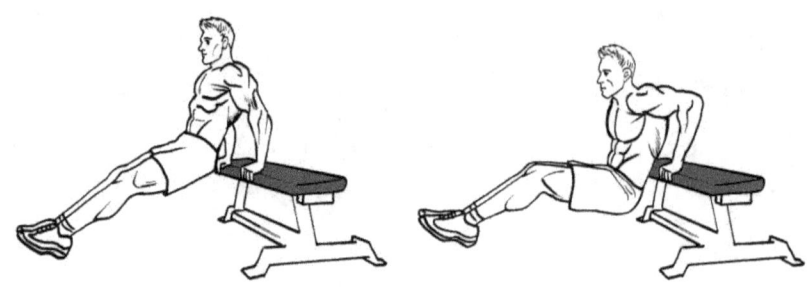

Starting position: Sit on flat bench perpendicular to your body. Put your arms behind you and to your sides and hold on to the edge of the bench with your hands. Now stick your legs out in front with a slight bend at the knee.

The exercise: Begin by pushing your torso up until your arms are locked out at the elbow joint and triceps flexed. Slowly lower your body by bending at the elbow joint until you lower yourself far enough to where there's 90 degrees between the upper arm and the forearm. Using your triceps to push your torso up, push your body back to the starting position.

Tip: Do not allow your torso to move away from the back of the bench. This can cause too much strain on the anterior head of the deltoids. Your back should lightly slide against the back of the bench as you're pushing your torso up and down during the exercise.

Muscles worked:

Primary: triceps

Secondary: anterior and lateral deltoids

Biceps

16. Standing BB curl

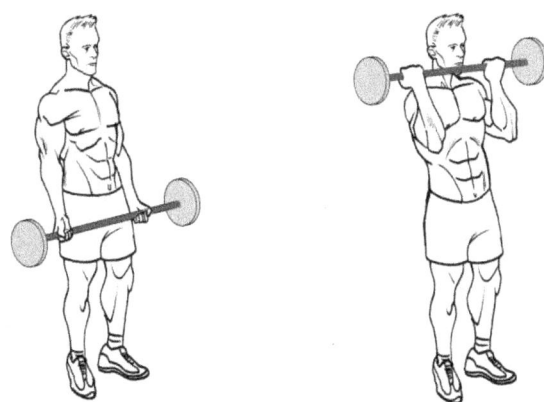

Starting position: Stand with feet about shoulder width apart holding a barbell with shoulder width grip. Keep your chest up and shoulders squared.

The exercise: Curl the weight up without leaning back, keeping your upper arms close to your sides, not allowing elbows to flare outward. Lower the weight down to starting position in a controlled manner.

Tip: Don't allow the torso to lean forward or backward in a swinging fashion while performing the exercise.

Muscles worked:

Primary: biceps, brachialis

Abdominals

17. Front plank

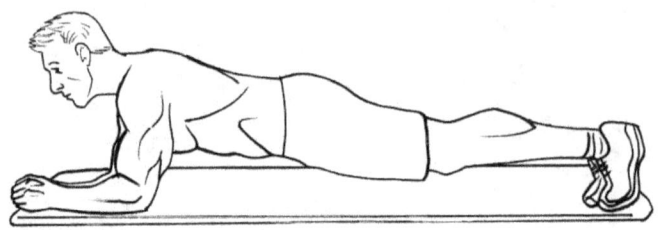

Starting position: Lie on your stomach with arms bent, palms and forearms on the ground, legs extended.

The exercise: Contract your ab muscles and slowly lift your entire torso off the floor, keeping palms, forearms, and toes on the ground. Avoid arching your lower back. Hold for up to one minute or shorter until strength increases.

Muscles worked:

Primary: rectus abdominis

Secondary: obliques, quadriceps, pectoralis major, serratus anterior

18. V-up crunch

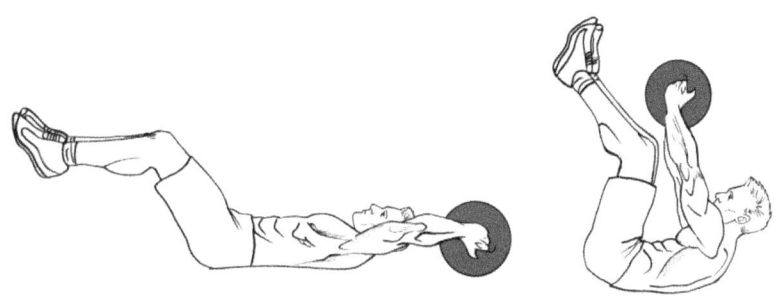

Starting position: Lay flat (supine) on mat with your feet together and your toes pointed toward the ceiling with hands on floor overhead and behind you.

The exercise: To begin the exercise, keep your legs straight and lift them up, and at the same time raise your upper body off of the floor and reach for your toes with your hands. Squeeze your abdominal muscles as you reach for your toes, and then slowly lower yourself back down to the starting position to finish the first repetition.

Tip: Begin each repetition with upper back on floor to allow abdominal muscles to work dynamically. The rectus abdominis and obliques contract only when actual waist flexion occurs. This is a rather difficult exercise to perform with good form and requires more coordination. To increase the difficulty, hold a medicine ball or weight plate behind your head.

Muscles worked:

Primary: rectus abdominis

Secondary: iliopsoas, obliques

19. Swiss ball crunches

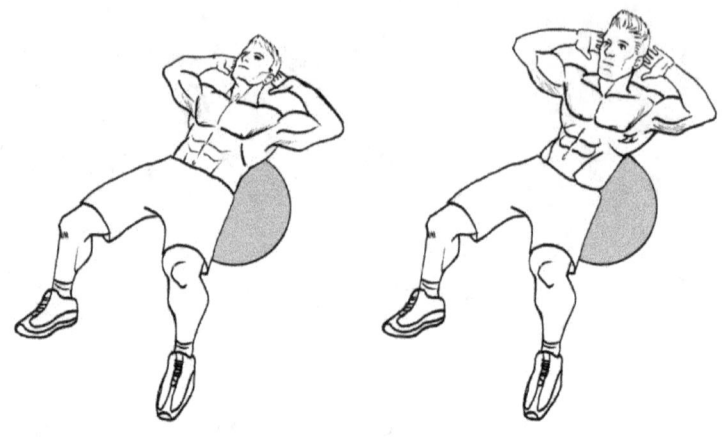

Starting position: Sit on a Swiss ball with your feet flat on the floor, shoulder width apart. Walk your feet forward as you lie back on the ball. Stop when the ball is under your hips, lower back, and middle back, knees bent 90 degrees.

Your lower back should feel like it's curved around the ball. Place your hands lightly behind your head and draw in your abs.

The exercise: Raise your chest up and slightly forward in a crunching motion. Do not pull on your neck to initiate the crunch. At the top of the movement, the middle of your back will lose contact with the Swiss ball. Now squeeze the abs and then slowly return to the starting position.

Muscles worked:

Primary: rectus abdominis

Secondary: obliques

About the Author

A master body transformation and nutrition coach, **Philip J. Hoffman** has studied the science behind fitness and nutrition all his life. He holds advanced degrees in biology, molecular biology and biochemistry. He has personally practiced his profession as a physique athlete since youth, and continues to rank in the top of the world for males over forty.

In his early career, he founded Body Image, a personal fitness training business to coach others reach their peak level of fitness. Today, he shares his gift more widely through HoffmanFit.com, authoring ebooks and leading his Online 12-Week Body Transformation Program. In addition, fitness enthusiasts benefit from his inaugural book, *The 9 Principles for a Lean and Defined Body*, which has earned hundreds of favorable Amazon reviews here in the U.S. and ranks near the top of Amazon Brazil in its category.

When this over-fifty father and entrepreneur isn't helping serious clients get fit and beautiful, he's modeling for commercial print ads in Los Angeles for some of the most recognized names in the industry.

HoffmanFit 12-Week Body Transformation Coaching Program

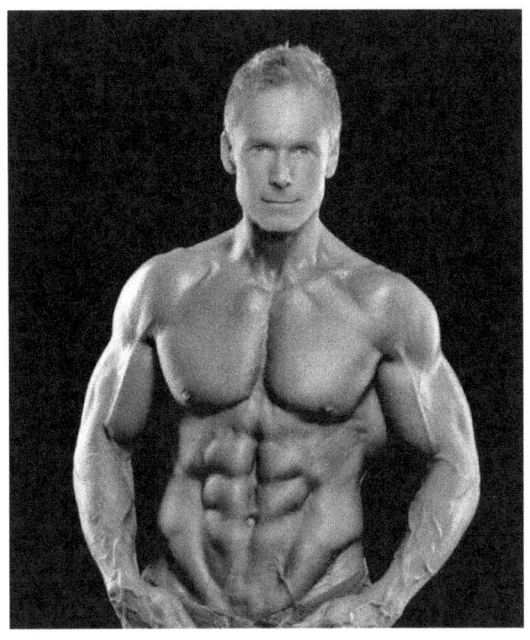

When is the time right?

Are you ready to get in the best shape of your life, even at middle age? Allow me to personally coach you in the most results-driven online 12-Week Body Transformation Program on the market. This is a no-nonsense, tried and proven approach. You will learn how to incorporate the fitness and nutrition system I've developed, which keeps me youthful and working as a fitness model and physique athlete — even at 50+ years young!

TO TRANSFORM YOUR BODY TODAY, GO TO: WWW.HOFFMANFIT.COM/TRANSFORMATION

 http://www.facebook.com/hoffmanfit

 http://www.pinterest.com/hoffmanfit